Published in 2015 b Publishing

Organic Guinea Pig'
Dale Preece-Kelly

All cover photography and artwork © 2015 Amanda Ravenall

The author asserts their moral right under the Copyright, Designs and Patents Act, 1988, to be identified as the author or authors of this work.

All Rights reserved. No part of this publication may be reproduced, copied, stored in a retrieval system, or transmitted, in any form or by any means, without the prior written consent of the copyright holder, nor be otherwise circulated in any form of binding or cover other than that in which it is published and without a similar condition being imposed on the subsequent purchaser.

A CIP catalogue record for this title is available from the British Library.

With thanks to my good friend Bobbi Capwell for her help deciding on a title

Dedicated to:

Gilly-Marie Harvey

my good friend & business partner in Organic Guinea Pig. She sowed the seed, and started me on the road to revolution, without her I never would have started questioning my lifestyle

AND

Kathryn Humphries

my best friend, my Butterfly Princess, the love of my life. She inspired me to take to the skies and fly myself, to spread the revolution. She was my "muse" whilst writing this book, and she will continue to be for my entire life. With all of my heart I dedicate this book to her – she saved my life

www.organicguineapig.com or find me on Twitter

CONTENTS

Introduction		Page 9
Chapter 1	Getting Started	Page 13
Chapter 2	Giving Up	Page 23
Chapter 3	Give Yourself Time	Page 47
Chapter 4	Increase Nutrients Replace Deficiencies	Page 52

Including Antioxidant Capacity Test

Chapter 5	A Question of Taste	Page 78
Chapter 6	The Role of Exercise	Page 89
Chapter 7	Positive Happiness	Page 106
Chapter 8	Juicing as a Refresher	Page 121
Chapter 9	Time to be Healthy (Or How to Avoid The Doc)	Page 137
Chapter 10	Maintaining The New You	Page 154
Chapter 11	Some Recipes to Get You Going	Page 167
	And Some Tips Too	Page 197

INTRODUCTION – Do you know who I am?

Well of course you don't, after all that is what introductions are all about isn't it? I certainly do hope, though, that at the end of this book you will know more about me, and want to find out even more by getting in touch!!

So what's the book about? I hear you ask. Imagine if I told you that I could show you a simple way to be a happier, healthier, fitter version of you. That I could show you a way to possibly reduce your medical costs, and to avoid the need to visit a doctor or take another pill again? To be happy every day, to live your dreams? Would that make you want to read more? Of course it would! Well I'm not here to guarantee that, but what you will get from this book are tools that will get you on the path to all of these things and more – these are just the side effects of taking back control of your life!

How rude! Please let me apologise, we haven't been introduced properly. My name is Dale Preece-Kelly, I am your author and I was the very first Organic Guinea Pig. I have a lot of firsts under my belt – for example, this is the first page of my first book and boy am I excited (not for the first time though!). What is an "Organic…..Guinea…..Pig"? Well, I have a friend and business partner who is also a nutritionist, and to prove to her that her advice helped people, and to give her the confidence to go out there and teach her message, I set up Organic Guinea Pig. Along the way OGP (as we shall call it) grew into something that today operates as a business in the UK, and is a lot more than just nutritional advice. What we teach is called OGP Lifestyle.

I am not trying to sell you my services, I am sharing what I teach with you in this book and if you've bought it, then you have taken the first step into a future that will hold undeniable freedoms for you and your body. You see when I began as the very first OGP, I was unhealthy – I smoked 15 to 20 cigarettes a day, I was drinking alcohol quite heavily (maybe a bottle of wine a night) I was eating badly, my mind was a scramble of ups and downs, my energy was low, I often felt depressed – the list goes on. The system I have followed since then, and am about to share with you, has led me to reverse all of that, and some of the side effects will blow you away, never mind what else it does for you.

You see what has happened is, I have come to realise that my body was controlling me – I would see a packet of chocolate biscuits and my hand would pick them up and put them into my shopping trolley, I would pick up a bottle of wine, and in it would go. This was my brain controlling my body, and giving in to the cravings that had developed from years of addiction to these wonderfully tasty treats. I felt that I needed to have these things in order to be happy, but did they make me happy? The answer, when I look back was "NO". What is happiness then? Happiness is being in CONTROL of your HQ (your brain) – Happiness is reclaiming the POWER to choose – Happiness is having the POWER to change. Because when you change certain things that you do, certain habits, replacing bad ones with good and when you change the way that you think about things, your WHOLE LIFE CHANGES!
When I took control, and began being mindful of what was happening around me all of the time, I lost weight,

my health improved, my body image improved both literally and mentally, my mental health improved, my positivity quota improved as did so much more. In short, my whole life improved. Come with me on the journey to your life's glorious future – take control and learn how to program your own sat nav for a better life and a better you…

Dale Preece-Kelly (www.organicguineapig.com)

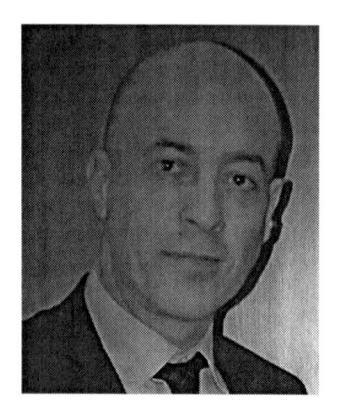

CHAPTER ONE – Getting Started

We are constantly bombarded with images of professionals and celebrities we trust, endorsing certain products – fizzy drinks, fast foods, junk foods, other lifestyle choices – this programs our brains to believe that these products are the ones to buy, what we need in order to be like them . . . this is lie #1. Our brains though, because they are currently in control of us, don't see it that way, our thought processes are all wrong. And this is the start of the spiral that takes us down to the realms of imbalance and disease.

Before we can take back control, we need to know where we are right now. We need a start point. My start point was being told by my doctor that I was headed for a third and fatal heart attack (I had my first 2 in 2010 - was this a wakeup call? Nope, my brain was still in control) – he told me that my blood pressure was dangerously, worryingly high, that my cholesterol was high and that I was a primary candidate for coronary disease and if I did not stop, DEATH! But my mind still insisted – it's OK, doctors ALWAYS blame cigarettes and alcohol. Being cynical about the medical profession anyway, I just figured he didn't really know what he was talking about and that my next check-in with him one month later would show that everything was fine.

I suffer with Parkinson's Disease, but have always managed to stave off symptoms without medication (I hate taking pills), but the symptoms had got worse than ever and I had to get pharmaceutical (hate that word too!) help to manage them too. I was a mess and mentally in a bad place too, and that's when I met Gilly – my current business partner in OGP, and one of two people who saved my life. She was big on nutrition, and raved at me passionately about organic food, especially fruit and vegetables. I think I was the first person to ever listen to her and tell her "You know what? Everything you are telling me is spot on. Where do I sign up?"

The next day, I went out and bought my first "healthy" grocery shop – I had been eating nothing but junk – mostly cheese rolls and fast food! I laid it all out on the counter and took a photograph of it, so proud of what I had done. This is how it looked:

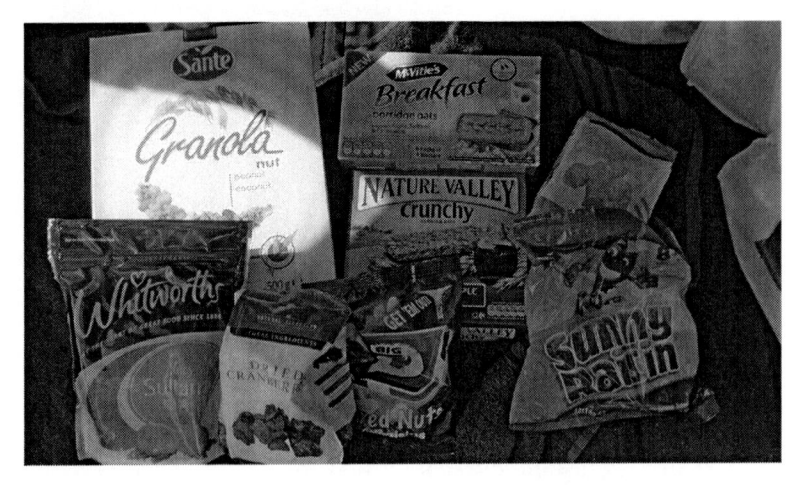

All processed foods – dried, manufactured, processed, preserved ... Bad for me. I did not look at the ingredients on the label, rather I used my perception from advertisements that I had read and seen of what was good for me. I sent this exact photograph to Gilly. She sent me a photo of the shop that she had just done, and then called me in hysterical laughter, unable to get over my perception of healthy. By the way, here is the photograph Gilly sent me:

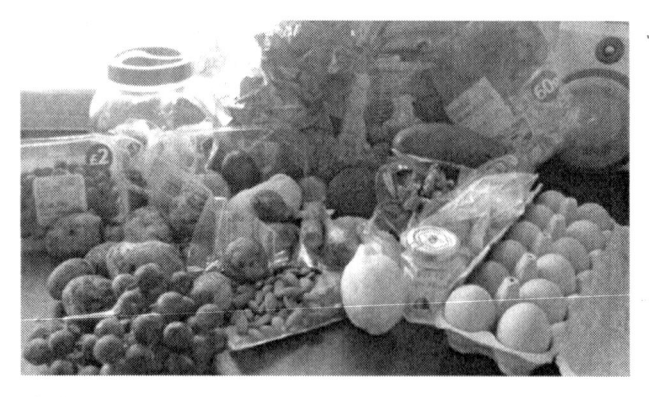

Much better, I am sure you agree. I would have bought this sort of thing to feed my pets, but not to feed me!! I was still a meat eater then, and ate many microwave meals – burgers, curries, pulled meats, all processed.

We call processed foods HIGH HI FOODS (HI = Human Interaction) which means that the food contained within has been through many people's hands from raw material to finished produce. What you see in the picture above is LOW HI FOODS (produce that has had little or NO human interaction from raw to plate). So that was my start point. You need one too. The first thing to do is go to your doctor (a complete contradiction you may think, but bear with me, because we are about to use our doctor in a completely different way – as our progress tester) – ask him to do simple tests, such as urine test, blood test, heart rate, blood pressure and weight, maybe even to measure your body mass index (or BMI) if you are overweight. Explain to them that you are about to initiate a healthy lifestyle change – and watch their horrified face appear! This is important for all sorts of reasons – firstly you need to make sure that your body can cope with what you are about to do to it, sometimes the body will resist us trying to change what it is used to! Secondly it is great to have a point to measure your progress against, because the next time you see them, if you follow what I am about to tell you, your readings will all be much improved !!! So we are using our doctor to independently monitor our health with our best interests at heart – after all, is that not why we pay them, they are in essence our employee, thus we are now controlling how THEY work for US?

We know where we are now, we have our starting point. The next thing you need to do is make a list of all of the "bad" or unhealthy things that you do. For instance, do you drink or smoke ; eat junk or sweets or chocolate ; live in a town or city ; drink soda or pop, coffee (with sugar and cream) or processed fruit juice ; look at what you do physically ; how you feel emotionally etc. Write it ALL down, you may be surprised at what you read afterwards, but you need an honest list, if you are going to control it all from now on. It's a scary thought and a big responsibility – so much easier to run on auto-pilot and not be responsible for the decision and choices you make when leading your lifestyle, but also a much faster decline in your quality of life. You see, with health and fitness comes happiness – and health is all about your environment (that's everything you eat, drink, do, breathe and think), if these are negative then your health is negative, your body reaches a tipping point where we are putting in too much bad stuff and we get imbalance, and this is when we see the symptoms of disease. When your environment is positive, is when we get balance and our health is positive too.

Now we want to know where we want to be when all of this pans out. At this point it is wise to set ourselves some goals. Do a 12 month plan, or a 24 month plan with simple, achievable goals. If you set the goals, then you are more likely to try and achieve them. If I were to say to you: "Your goal for month one is to eat NO chocolate at all", well you may just take out a chocolate bar and put the whole thing in your mouth! None of us likes being told what to do by others, especially when it comes to things that we are doing that we enjoy. So set your own goals, but they MUST be realistic, simple and achievable.

You may decide that all you want to do in month 1 is quit smoking – I did it in a day – 4th July 2014. I got in my car and was on my last smoke in the pack. I put it in my mouth and I lit up. I had been thinking about quitting for a while, as I had started to dislike the taste. I took a deep drag, and said to myself: "Dale, this is your final cigarette. You will buy no more, you will smoke no more, this is the end!" Was it easy? No it was not, but we shall talk about this in the next chapter – Chapter 2 – Giving Up.

It may be easier to list all of the things you are prepared to do without to begin with and start that way, moving on to everything else once you have achieved the first few. Or you may just want to blitz them all, and completely overhaul your life and get that better you faster. Whatever you decide, the changes you make will be permanent and easily maintained, because you will have that one thing that will keep you going . . . COMMITMENT! If you are 100% committed to doing something then it will always happen.

Finally, now you have your list of goals, I want you to write your ultimate goal on a piece of A4 paper in large colourful letters. It should be a simple statement, that will become your mantra, your driving force, your reason for commitment . . . it may be to drop 3 dress sizes, or to drop 50 pounds or to live long enough to see your grandkids grow up, to get rid of those little niggly health problems you have (did I mention that what I am about to tell you can also revolutionise your health, in terms of helping to prevent and relieve symptoms of disease? In some cases it even takes the symptoms and the diseases away completely!) Whatever it is write it down, but write it in a way that makes it a positive affirmation, using words like WILL and CAN, for example "I WILL drop three dress sizes by July 2016" or "I CAN lose 50 pounds and be healthy". Now laminate it and put it somewhere you will see it clearly and for a long time each day – it may be on your kitchen notice board, on the counter, on the wall next to the tv, on your bedroom mirror.

Each time you see that note, it will act as a motivator, reminding you why you are putting yourself through all of the withdrawal and the cold turkey – that's right many of our bad habits are addictions, and you will crave them, but that note is there to remind you why you should NOT give in to those cravings. Each time you look at it, I also want you to repeat it out loud to yourself ~ "I want to live long enough to see my grandkids grow up" ~ even if it's 20 times a day, no matter who is there with you. Don't feel silly; feel confident, because you WILL do this.

This won't all happen overnight, it will happen gradually, and it's better that way. Hopefully as you work your way through this book you will begin to make subtle changes as you realise the actions you need to take. These changes are the beginnings of regaining control of your life. No it won't happen overnight, it will take time (depending on your current state it could take up to 2 years) but over the course of your reading this book, and by the time you get to the end of it, you will start to feel happier and feel good that you have taken your life back into YOUR OWN hands and made a start on your journey to a better you.

You are already one step further forward ~ "Stick with me, the best is yet to come"

CHECKLIST:
1. Visit doctor for a check-up
2. Make a list of everything I eat, drink, do, breathe and think that is unhealthy
3. Make a monthly "Goal List" for the next 12 to 24 months – goals must be simple, realistic and achievable.
4. Write down your ULTIMATE Goal, as a positive affirmation, laminate and post it somewhere it will be seen by you many times a day

CHAPTER TWO – Giving Up

Any lifestyle change requires sacrifices to be made. Let me define that more clearly, because I am stating that giving up something that is inherently unhealthy for us constitutes a sacrifice! The sacrifices you are making, what you are sacrificing, are those things that you THINK make you happy. These are habits and habits take time to change – time we shall discuss in the next chapter. Let me show you what I mean – these are the sacrifices that I have made so far on my journey:

- Cigarettes
- Bread and related products
- Fast food (fish & chips, McDonalds, KFC etc.)
- Coffee
- Dairy products
- Biscuits
- Some alcohol
- Meat
- Sweets
- Chocolate

- Sugars

Not that I am saying you have to give all of these things up. Some of these I chose to give up (such as meat and dairy) and others I needed to give up for my health. These things have all been replaced with the sacred fruit and vegetables, nuts, seeds and pulses.

Giving up some of these things is easy; giving up others is so tough it's scary! Do you have to never eat your favourite unhealthy foods never again? Not at all, and later in this chapter we shall introduce you to the "Freedom Mentality" ~ something which, if you are disciplined enough, will allow you to have the odd treat. Whatever you give up will be hard, because it is already such a big part of your life that it needs to be "given up". You will go through "cold turkey", there will be mood swings, there may be tears, you may shake, get stomach cramps – a lot of these foods are like drugs, and you will need strong willpower (something we shall address later). There are others you will give up with ease, because you will immediately feel so much better from not having them, that you will not want them again.

So let's take each one of them in turn, but first it must be stated that it would be impossible to give up all of these things at the same time and in the same way as I did, we are all YOU-nique and all need to address quitting in the best way that suits us. The easiest way to fail would be to stop everything at the same time – like climbing a mountain, giving up has to be done gradually and if done in the right way, the summit can be reached. Here they are:

Smoking – This was a tough one for me, and the first thing I gave up. I was smoking 15-20 per day.
I have tried a number of times in the past to quit, using patches, gum, inhalers etc but always lapsed back. The longest I had previously gone was 3 weeks. After being told by a doctor that I was heading for a fatal heart attack unless I gave up a number of things, including cigarettes, I was in denial. I am a little cynical of the medical profession, and they quite often blame smoking and drinking for a multitude of ailments, and so I waved my hand dismissively and carried on doing what I was doing.

One day, I was leaving my work in a secure psychiatric hospital, with just one cigarette left in my pack. I got in my car and lit up. I had not been enjoying the taste for a while, but it was my only real vice and so it wasn't easy to let it go. As I took a deep drag on my last cigarette, and I said to myself (out loud) "That's it, no more. I will buy no more, I will smoke no more". And that was that, I did not buy any more! That was until a month later, when I got dumped! This was the stress that drove me back to it – I bought and smoked a pack of 10 over a weekend, but I knew that by buying them I was not going to start again, it was a temporary hiatus. I chose to smoke that pack and no more. And I am happy to say that I have not smoked a cigarette since that weekend. I was determined to give up smoking and because of that determination it worked – you have to really want it! In terms of reaction to giving up – I had cravings for them and for other food, I had mood swings – especially frustration and anger, I had the shakes. In addition, when I gave up smoking I developed a nasty cough for the first 7 – 10 days, but it soon left me, I got mouth ulcers, I even got a couple of colds in the first 28 days, as smoking dampens your immune system and as the toxins leave your body, this is how they do it! I really wanted to continue my hourly habit of putting one of those things in my mouth and filling my lungs with poison (we do this out of choice), but I resisted. I just kept reminding myself that I really did not like the way that they tasted, and that helped stop me asking for a pack when I was standing at a counter facing the rack of cigarette choice! When I initially stopped, it took about a week for these feelings to leave me, my little hiatus a month later caused no problems at all and I just stopped and carried on as I was.

It does help to develop other habits. I have since learned that eating celery takes away nicotine cravings (make a note of that one!), its taste is not dissimilar and the phytonutrients contained within the vegetable help to replace some of the chemicals related to the craving at the same time as helping your body to heal from the effects of smoking. I concentrated on how long it took for the craving for a cigarette to deplete – it took about 10 minutes for me, but may take a little longer or a little less time for you – it was about the length of time it takes from the need to have one to having finished smoking. So you need something to do for those 10 minutes. I would flick through Facebook and Twitter, or read a book for 10 minutes, to take my mind off it, and I found that it really worked. Once I started that distraction, the need to smoke just went. At the end of the day, all it is is a habit – a habit that kills you, but it's just a habit that serves no other purpose. Some say it calms them down or helps them relax – nope – it's immediate effect is as a stimulant, on account of it releasing adrenaline into the bloodstream, and is both physically and psychologically addictive, hence the reason why people find it so hard to kick the habit. However, because people THINK it calms them down, they believe it, and it becomes an EXCUSE for smoking.

So if you want to quit smoking, just quit! If you have a heavy habit – i.e. you smoke more than 20 a day, then you will need to cut down gradually – by 10 a week, which means it may take a few weeks to finally be smoke free. I was on 15-20 per day and I just stopped, and it took immense willpower – however, I am an extremely positive person and that helps, as did the fact that I really wanted to quit. Oh, and remember celery – eating celery instead of smoking a cigarette! It stops the craving, but it's also great for your blood pressure and therefore you are already starting to repair your body as you quit. I would not recommend e-cigs or vaping, as that just reinforces the habit of smoking (i.e. something is in your fingers, and you are repeatedly putting it to your mouth and inhaling, just like smoking a cigarette) and patches and gum did not work for me.

Willpower is discussed later in this chapter, so please refer to that section if you need help in that area. As you will find out later on in this chapter my willpower was useless against some of my more favourite "habits"!

Bread, Cakes & Related Products – This one was pretty easy for me. You know that bloated feeling you get when you eat heavy doughy foods, and you feel really full, and your tummy distends abnormally? The cause is yeast, which feeds candida in the gut – this is a fungus that builds up and never goes away. Many people are actually allergic to the proteins in wheat that we know as gluten (a gluey substance that remains when flour is washed to remove the starch) and this causes the reaction in the gut that we know as bloating. If you want that feeling to go away then the answer is simple – STOP eating it! If you want to eat bread on occasion, then do it under the "Freedom Mentality". I still eat bread VERY occasionally, and do not have the problems I used to associate with eating these products, because I do it under the freedom mentality and do not over indulge.

Fast Food (Fish & Chips, McDonalds, KFC etc.) – Deep fried and fatty foods are tough to give up, because they taste so good. We love our staple fish and chips, fried chicken, fries from the local burger joint, some even love deep fried chocolate bars! However, eating deep fried foods is incredibly bad for you. This is not saying that you cannot or must not eat deep fried foods; it means that you really should not. Freedom Mentality, though, allows us to CHOOSE what we eat and when we eat it, in the knowledge that we are allowing ourselves to do it as an exception, and that's ok. After reading this you may not choose to eat it at all.

When oil used for deep frying (olive oil, sunflower oil etc.) is heated to above 200/250 degrees, it loses any goodness it may have had and produces FREE RADICALS – these are unstable molecules, that damage or injure the healthy cells in your body by stealing their electrons to stabilise themselves – this damages the DNA of the healthy cells, causing disease. Hot oil also produces carcinogens, which are the nasty's that lead to the formation of cancer cells.

So think about that for a few seconds. Is that enough to make you think twice about eating deep fried food? If not, then read on some more.

Let me tell you a story - I decided after Christmas, that I would eat nothing but healthy foods. It was supposed to be a 28 day juicing "detox", however, as it was so cold it was tough to maintain. What I therefore did was drink 3 juices per day, and then in the evening have a nice hot and hearty homemade soup, made with fresh organic ingredients. About 22 days in, I was out on the road working, and had a 2 hour break between bookings. I went to park up (in my usual place) but there were no spaces, and I therefore found somewhere else to park. I ended up outside a chip shop – the produce smelt beautiful, you know that smell that just draws you in? So in I went and bought myself a small cone of chips . . . I ate them, I enjoyed them, and they were nice. About 5 minutes afterwards I got that feeling in my stomach, the one where you know that your body is going to reject the contents. Not good. So on went my sat nav, and I found my nearest supermarket, so that I could use a toilet. I was violently ill – within minutes my body had realised that I was putting bad stuff into it and rejected it in the worst possible way.

My body, and I guess my brain to some extent, had been reprogrammed to a healthier lifestyle, and had become accustomed to being sustained with healthy nutrition and was telling me in no uncertain terms that my lapse was not acceptable. Strange how you do these things without thinking or realising. Just by feeding my body the right foods for 20 days, I had taught it what was right for it, and it told me when I made an error of judgement. Now when I smell that smell or get that urge to eat deep fried foods, all I have to do is to recall that memory, and remind myself that my body does not (a) like me to feed it deep fried foods (b) like the effects caused by deep fried foods. That memory takes away the desire to eat these foods. It's great to be able to associate a bad habit with a bad experience, as it stops the desire to do the habit to a certain extent.

Sweet Sugary Foods – (Please note that this refers to PROCESSED sugars, NOT natural sugars, that you may find in fruit and veg – these work in a totally different way)

Not such an easy one to deal with, this one. Sugar is one of the most highly addictive additives in food. Sugar cane or beet is highly processed to make granulated white sugar. This is potent and easily absorbed into the body, which cause a rise in insulin levels, which in turn raises the endorphin (feel good hormones) levels, which causes the body to have a chemical high. Continuously feeding your body with these foods eventually causes the natural endorphin level to slow in order to regulate the flow of endorphins to the brain. Once the flow of endorphins slows, we don't feel so happy (or high) and this can lead to depression – so we eat more sweet sugary foods, to get more endorphins etc. etc. – it's a vicious circle of eating and drinking, which leads to us becoming obese.

When we go for the "sugar free" or "diet" option, in order to avoid the obesity problems and addictive nature, we are consuming other chemicals which substitute the processed sugars. Whilst these chemicals are calorie free, they are even worse for us than sugar!

One of these chemicals is called ASPARTAME – it is a chemical used to coat the space shuttle, it melts Teflon, it is carcinogenic, and proven to cause other diseases too (such as Parkinson's Disease). It was discovered by mistake by a scientist, as an artificial sweetener, and initially WAS NOT granted approval for use in foods by the FDA. The WORST thing about aspartame is that it makes the body CRAVE carbohydrates, which in turn lead to obesity – so by consuming food and drinks (such as diet sodas) laced with aspartame as an artificial sweetener, you are actually INCREASING your risk of obesity!!! The saying is "Aspartame puts the DIE into DIET!" Beware too, because aspartame also goes under a few other names.

The trick is to avoid "sugar free" and "diet" foods and drinks at all lengths possible. They just lead to more illness and disease or make current ailments worse. It does not matter who makes them, or who advertises them, the ingredients and effects are standard across the board.

We have a great food processor attached to us, it's called the body – we have a mouth that chews up the ingredients and a digestive system that processes them in the most effective way for our body. If we put good, healthy, organic ingredients into our mouths and allow the body to process them, we know what has gone into our food, and we know exactly how it has been processed. When we eat processed foods, we do not know how they have been made or how they have been processed. Go to your freezer now and take out one of those ready meals and read the ingredients…..it will have sugar in it (heavily processed sugar) and a number of ingredients that we are not familiar with. Do the same with a bag of sweets, or a chocolate bar, or a cake. Get used to reading ingredients lists – the higher the ingredient is on the list, the higher the content of that ingredient within the food. Sugar is normally either the first or second ingredient on the list!!!

If you know people who work in food processing plants, ask them if they eat the food their plant processes. Chances are that their answer will be a big fat negatory!!

A good way to get a sweet but wholesome snack or meal or pudding, is to look for foods containing a natural sugar – FRUIT! Fruits like blueberries, strawberries, raspberries, cherries and grapes, for example, make lovely sweet snacks that will not only satiate your need for a sweet snack, but will also deliver great healthy vitamins, minerals, nutrients and antioxidants to your body's bloodstream at the same time. Substituting your refined sugar intake, with the natural unprocessed fructose (sugar found in fruit) can also help to prevent the risks of cancer. You will always see or hear the argument from people that the sugar found in fruit is just as bad for you if not worse than refined sugars – this is a complete fallacy. You see, instead of breaking down fructose rapidly (as happens with refined sugars), the body processes it more slowly allowing the "high" to happen progressively and naturally. Also once your diet consists of healthy foods, drinks and snacks (all natural, not out of a box or carton), your body reacts favourably – you find you have more energy, a better metabolic rate, you have good skin, you are happier, and you generally feel on top of the world EVERY single day, like you can handle anything life throws at you!!

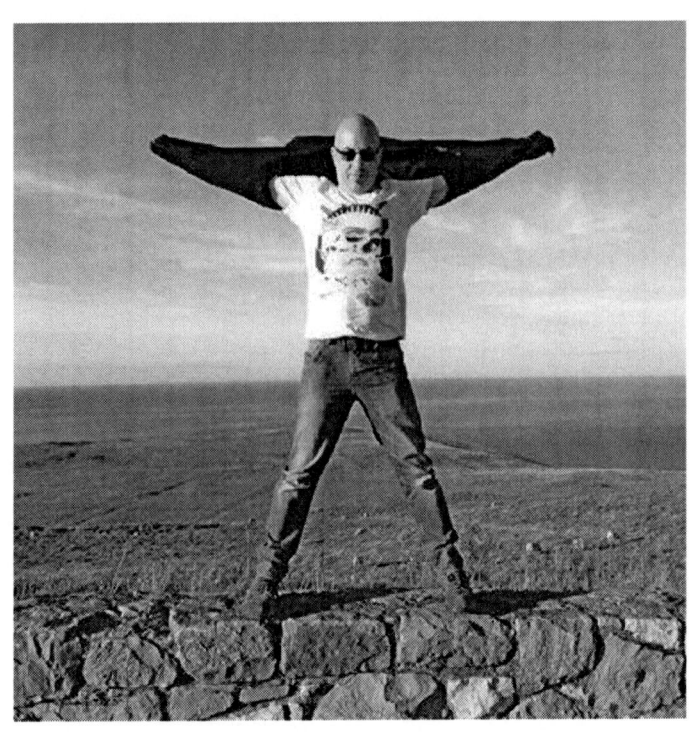

If chocolate is one of your downfalls, then look for recipes that use natural raw cacao (NOT cocoa) – this is the healthiest, purest form of chocolate you can consume, and is minimally processed. Cacao is thought to be a food that is the highest source of antioxidants and magnesium of ALL foods. (There is a recipe at the end of this book for healthy chocolate orange brownies). The internet is full of healthy options, with recipes using cacao and many other healthy foods, for making healthy snacks that will satisfy your need for sweets, candy, chocolate and other sweet foods. All we need to do is embrace our desire to be healthy and open our eyes, to see what is there for us all.

Everything Else – the above 4 items are the ones we really need to try and give up if we want to give ourselves the best chance at becoming healthier, happier and fitter. The rest of the foods I listed, that I gave up, were given up out of choice:

Meat – I had wanted to be vegetarian for a long time, but my previous lifestyle and relationship meant that had I done so, I would have alienated myself from friends and family. I was forced into eating foods that I did not really enjoy, nor ethically agree with, because of the circles of people that I lived in. The end of a relationship and a move of region, allowed me to change the way that my entire lifestyle operated. My love for animals and passion for their welfare, my lack of interest in eating meat and my newfound passion for food and phytonutrients, superfoods, antioxidants, vitamins and minerals - all gained naturally - allowed me to become vegetarian. I have never looked back, nor have I for one single millisecond craved meat.

PLANTS HAVE PROTEIN TOO YOU KNOW!

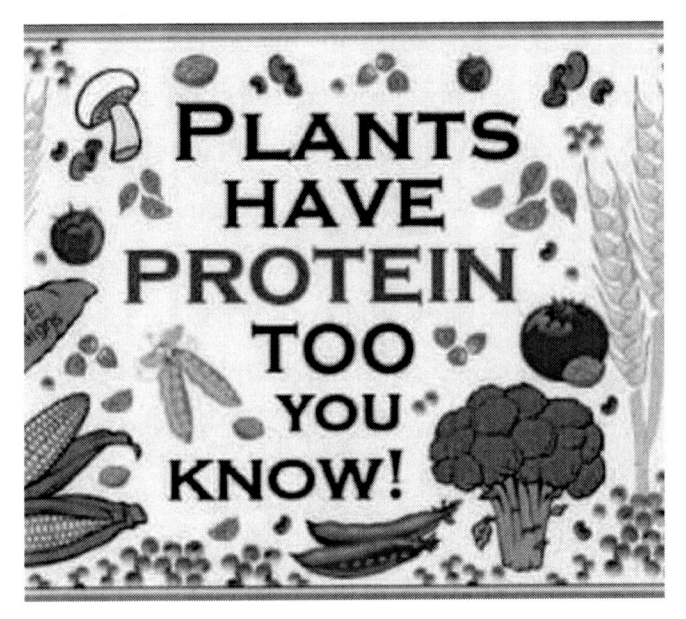

As a vegetarian, I am asked all of the time: "Where do you get your protein from?" – Well this is the answer I give to them. "Plants have protein too you know" - many of the foods I eat contain proteins, and sometimes in higher quantities than meat. Foods such as greens (broccoli, kale, spinach), nuts, seeds, beans and grains for example make great sources of protein.

Dairy Products – I no longer drink animal milk in any way shape or form, I prefer to use nut milks such as almond milk or coconut milk. Something I do still eat, however, is cheese, but I have found that my tastes have changed. I used to be able to put away one pound of cheese in about 5 days, usually mature cheddar, nowadays though my cheese consumption is probably not even a pound a month!! I also will eat cheeses that I have never eaten before, such as halloumi and feta.

Again, giving up dairy products was not a tough thing to do, I just stopped and do not really miss it. I find that my digestive complaints have disappeared completely with the loss of wheat (gluten) and dairy products from my diet – no more bloating, no more indigestion, no more reflux, no more digestive problems at all!!

Finally Coffee – Coffee has not completely gone from my life, but it is now a choice through freedom mentality, rather than a lifestyle. To put it into perspective, I was drinking 6 cups plus of coffee a day; now I drink 1-2 cups of coffee per month!! This is something that I always craved – like cigarettes – but something that I no longer craved. Caffeine is another drug (like nicotine) that we have trouble leaving behind – we get cravings, some people get the shakes, other people become bad tempered. Once the body has cleared the caffeine in its system (takes about 3-5 days), however, life becomes a lot easier. These days, I start the day with a mug of warm filtered water containing a slice of lemon and a slice of ginger – lemons are a natural energiser, hydrating and oxygenating the body, making it feel revitalised and refreshed and ginger sets the stomach up to receive food. I drink a couple of litres a day – it's like drinking water, but with added benefits!

Does this give me the boost that caffeine gave me? Partly. For the rest of the boost, along with my mug of warm filtered water with lemon and ginger, I take a shot . . . . Yes, you did read that right!! My shot is either, pineapple & ginger, apple & ginger or lime, ginger & chili!!! It makes a shot glass full of juice, and like a shot you down it in one, but it is like having a triple espresso in terms of the NATURAL boost you get from it.

Oh and if you drink decaffeinated coffee, you aren't helping yourself either! When coffee beans are turned into coffee they are processed, to decaffeinate it the already processed coffee has to be processed further. They use chemicals to remove as much caffeine as they can, generally 97% of it. These chemicals can cause problems in our bodies too; in addition antioxidants found naturally in the coffee bean are even further destroyed in the decaffeination process. If you must drink coffee, then buy the raw unprocessed beans, and then process them yourself by filtering – this way you retain most of the antioxidants present.

Now let's talk about Freedom Mentality and Willpower:

Freedom Mentality
Freedom mentality is what we are hoping to give you with this book – the freedom to choose, as oppose to the restriction of "CAN'T". The "can't" mentality breeds contempt and resentment. The freedom mentality means being able to eat what you want when you want without the resentment or guilt of the "can't mentality". Freedom mentality gives you back control – the POWER of choice. You choose to have the chocolate bar, because you CAN and it's fine, because it's a one off. The "can't" mentality would allow you to have the chocolate bar, but the difference is it wouldn't stop there!! With a freedom mentality, you can apply the 80/20 rule (I prefer to use an 85/15 or a 90/10) – so long as 80% of the time you are eating and drinking,

thinking and doing in a mindfully conscious and healthy way, then you will be much happier, fitter and healthier than you are today. It's all about being mindful of what you are doing, and making conscious decisions to do the right thing – taking back control of your life requires you to apply the "Freedom Mentality" and be conscious in everything you do.

Willpower

Willpower - control of one's impulses and actions; self-control.

Let me tell you the story of how I discovered the secret of WILLPOWER:

Willpower is a funny old thing, but I think I have finally figured out how it works . . . sometimes it seems you have it and sometimes it feels like it's escaped, however I have come to realise it is ALWAYS there you just have to allow it to present itself, and not hold it back.

Will Power is the name of the little angel sitting on your shoulder - today he spoke to me and I recognised him. I love my biscuits, and at times when I am hungry or fancy a snack, and go into a shop I find it really hard to resist those sweet chocolatey biscuity treats - today I bought a banana, thanks to Will!!

I stopped at the plain chocolate digestives (my real Achilles) which were on sale at £1 a pack and I stood for a few minutes, freedom mentality telling me it was ok to have them (but this was just a ruse, the other fella using my new found control mechanism against me). Then I walked down to the fruit and picked up a banana, because Will reminded me that I had been craving one for days (I hadn't been craving the biscuits or chocolate, I really had been craving a healthy snack – a banana) and therefore it would satisfy me more than the processed sweet snack, and I knew that it would stave off the hunger for much longer.

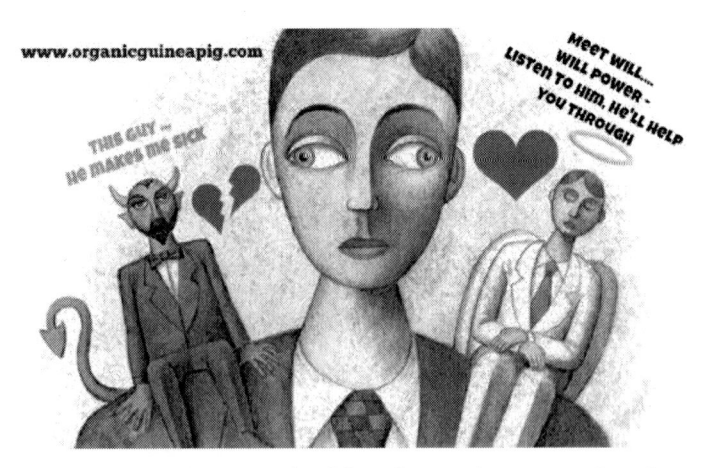

I then went BACK to the biscuits, and contemplated some more, but Will told me to look at my left hand - there was my banana - logic and reason could not convince me that I wanted the chocolate biscuits any more. I went with just a banana to the till and paid for it - 25p. Not only did I take the healthy option, but in addition I saved 75p!! WIN / WIN.

Self control, sounds easy, but it's not. It is the retraining of your mind to perform a different action from that which you are used to performing. You brain is in control of your bodily functions, which include asking for those cigarettes, picking up a chocolate bar, walking into McDonalds, filling your shopping basket or trolley with sweet sugary items and processed foods like crisps, biscuits and sweets. When we change our lifestyle, we need to take back control from our brain, so we can train our mind (the part of our brain which allows us to think, reason and CHOOSE) to think in a different way – reprogram it if you like, so that when our brain says "pick up that bar of chocolate", we reply by saying "well as much as I know it would taste good, and I CAN have it, I don't want it". This is our "Freedom Mentality"

At first it looks weird to other shoppers – you are in the biscuit aisle, stopped, surveying the produce, your hand reaches out, and then retracts, and then reaches out again, and retracts again, and then off you walk! You do get to the point, though, where you just walk straight down the aisle without stopping. This is when your "mind training" is completed, you are free of your addiction, you have GIVEN UP!

If you need help with your thought processes, willpower and support then please use the contact details in the introduction.

"Without excuses, ANYTHING is possible"

CHAPTER THREE – Give Yourself Time

"Rome wasn't built in a day." I don't know about you, but that was a common theme from my parents growing up. You see, I don't have the most amazing patience threshold in the world; in fact, I would go so far as to say that my impatience knows no bounds. If I decide that I want something, then I have to have it NOW! If I order something online, then I want it tomorrow! As we all know though, life does not happen like that.

My transformation has not happened overnight and, to be fair, you don't want it to – you see gradual is sustainable. If you tried to go from being a 20 stone couch potato to an 11 stone athlete, and you started on a Monday and wanted to go show your new body off on the beach at the weekend, then you would be sorely disappointed. My transformation happened – incidentally it's still happening, but we're talking majority here, what I am now working at (as I write this book) are the icing and the cherry on the cake (if you will pardon the reference) – in around 7 months. That's two thirds of a year! As I say, it is still going on, but I am through the biggest part and now honing it so that I am (a) healthy and (b) fit. Happiness and positivity are two of the side effects of leading a healthy lifestyle.

So how long realistically can you expect it to take you? 7 months in and I was still battling sugar cravings – cravings for biscuits and sweets. I've never really been one for eating chocolate bars and cakes, or craving them, chocolate bars were something I really had to want to buy them, and I preferred biscuits and sweets. These were the things that really took some willpower to resist; I would have to say that they took MAXIMUM willpower.

From this experience and information, I would have to say that sugary foods are probably the hardest processed food to give up. So what did I do to curb the cravings for sugary foods? Well I did use "freedom mentality", but knowing that this was my processed food Achilles Heel, "freedom mentality" was me just giving myself permission to eat them – not just once in a while (as "freedom mentality" dictates) but most days. Sometimes I would go for a few days without, but then I would see something and tell myself it was ok. How did I then beat the draw of sweets and biscuits, and the freedom of being able to choose when all that was in my head was the CAN'T (Constant And Never-ending Tantrum) mentality of : well I want it but I CAN'T have it, and that's just not fair!

I used fruit! Fruit I enjoyed – grapes and strawberries, melon and pineapple, apples and more. This meant that I could carry with me in my car (when working or travelling long distances) a juice, usually an orange one, as these are my favourite – generally made with apples and carrots. I also carry fruits such as apples and bananas which have plenty of insoluble fibre which is filling. Fruits can also be bought from any supermarket or local shop too, usually for less than a packet of biscuits or bag of sweets.

In addition, if I want more than one flavour, I eat health food snacks – these can be bought from your local health food store. Just check those ingredients first to ensure that they are made purely with wholefoods, without any chemical additives or preservatives.

In terms of time for a full transformation, well you need to give yourself at least a good 12 to 18 months. In this time, though, you are constantly improving little by little in terms of health, fitness, happiness. You are getting better and better and you are changing habits. Habits are tough cookies to crack (I seem to be using a few processed food metaphors in this book!), and it is widely known that a bad habit takes around 28 days to change to a good habit, some take longer and some take less – it depends on the individual.

What you need to do, is to start with the really bad habits such as smoking and drinking soda/pop, and then you have started working on two aspects of becoming a better you: your health and your nutritional intake. Stopping these two alone will start making you feel like a better you in just 7-14 days – in that time you will be able to breathe better (although when you give up smoking you will develop a cough and may get ulcers and colds, as smoking dampens your immune system and as the toxins leave your body, this is how they do it), you will have more energy, your cravings for food should die down and you may even begin to see a drop in your weight!

This in turn will make you feel happier and healthier and should give you motivation to continue. The more bad stuff that you give up, the better you will feel. The more positive things you do for yourself, the less you will crave the bad stuff, the more motivated you will be and the better you will feel. Every day a little better!!

"Every journey of a thousand miles, begins with a single step" ~ Lao Tzu

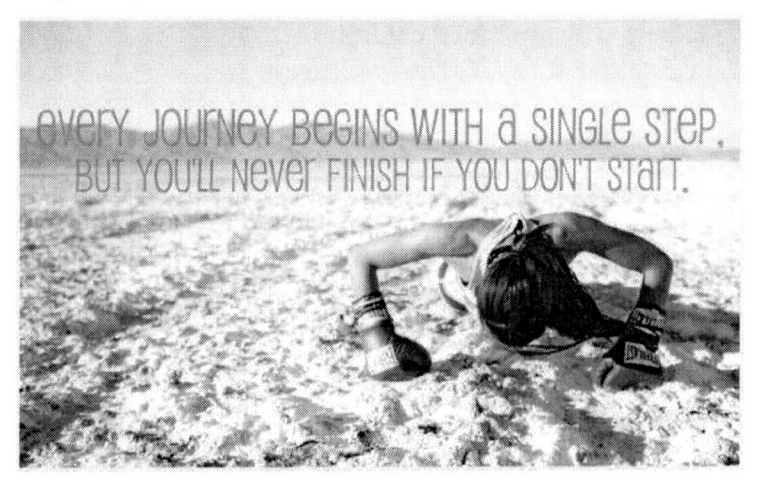

CHAPTER FOUR – Increase Nutrients Replace Deficiencies

In this chapter, I hope to give you a basic knowledge of which foods are the healthiest. I cannot explain in the space that I have everything that I have learned in my training as a Nutritional Therapist, but I am going to try to help with your food choices.

The biggest question to ask is "What are the healthiest foods?" As you saw in Chapter One, my idea of healthy came from the adverts I had seen in magazines and on TV of foods promoted as "healthy" by celebrities!! I knew nothing about what to look for on ingredient lists or even how they worked. Things have changed since then and I have developed a good knowledge of how ingredient lists work, as well as knowing which foods are GREAT for repairing my cells, so that I look as good on the inside as I do on the outside.

Ingredient Lists

As a starting point let's talk about processed foods and ingredients lists. If possible remove processed foods from your diet completely! We are blessed with the best food processing equipment known to man – our mouths and our stomachs – and if we know what we are putting into our bodies, then we can make a fair assessment of how it is going to affect our body. You see, processed foods contain all manner of different chemicals which help to enhance flavours and colours, and help to preserve the food that is inside the box. Not all countries carry laws that make manufacturers list all ingredients or indeed where they come from. In the USA for instance, manufacturers do not have to label that ingredients are from a genetically modified source – in the UK, however, they do. Please bear this in mind. Basic rules of reading ingredient lists:

- If you cannot pronounce the ingredient – then don't buy it.
- Ingredients are listed with the highest content ingredient first, therefore if sugar or fat are high

up on the list then chances are it is not a healthy choice, as you will be loading your body with sugars and fats. Sugar is often listed second on a lot of processed foods.
- If chemicals – i.e. E numbers, those long words that are difficult to pronounce, flavourings, preservatives etc. – are high up on the list then it's not a healthy choice, as you will simply be loading your body with chemicals.

Even look at the ingredients on liquids, you may be surprised – for instance diet sodas and diet cordials will contain aspartame (there is that word again!) or a derivative that is essentially a poison! If it is not listed then check the country of origin, as it may not be a requirement in that country to list such ingredients. Low fat options are also a bad idea – these will contain chemicals to make the food taste the same or similar to the full fat version (even those from the diet clubs that are manufactured as part of their regimes and are advertised by celebrities as the ones to eat). Make the choice to go for the version that has not been meddled with chemically.

As we said in the previous chapter, you cannot do all of this at once, and so there will be a transitional time when you are moving from processed foods to healthy alternatives, where you are starting to cut down on processed foods. Whilst going through this period, go for the full fat and full sugar food and drink alternatives. Eat butter NOT margarine – it is commonly known that margarine is just one molecule away from being plastic! Butter although it is fatty, is 100% naturally made and not processed. You can also make your own, from nuts. Dairy is not as healthy as we are led to believe, either - fresh unpasteurised milk is straight from the cow, it is then pasteurised (process one), then it is processed again to become the semi-skimmed version (process two), then it is processed once more to become the skinny or zero or full-skimmed option (process three and maybe even four) – therefore I will let you decide for yourself which is the best choice to make! Again you can make your own nut milk, which is delicious – more about this later.

So you see, it's all about the ingredients, and you can tell a lot about a processed food from its list of ingredients. Be wary, whatever it is you are buying, because a lot of time just a glance at that list is enough to make you put it back on the shelf. Even when we are told it is healthy, once we start to look at what is contained in the food or drink, we realise that it really is not. The thing is, a lot of us believe what we are told by adverts and "trusted" manufacturers and never think to question it – only when we have the knowledge of what we are dealing with, and how it affects our body, do we begin to sit up and ask questions. The purpose of this book is to arm you with that knowledge and give you answers to some of those questions. You can then make educated and informed decisions to improve your health and improve your life.

Foods without Ingredients Lists

"Foods without ingredients lists?" I hear you ask. Yes, they do exist! We call them Low Human Interaction Foods – the best type, as an example, is an apple that you have picked off the tree yourself. If all you do before you decide on a food is ask yourself "Is this Low Human Interaction or High Human Interaction food?" and then put the Low HI Food in your basket and the High HI Foods back on the shelf, then this book has done its job in some way – it's made you think about what you are putting into your body.

So, foods that do not need to list their ingredients are fresh whole foods, which are not processed at all. If a nut is out of its shell and bagged, then it needs an ingredients list (and it will also carry the allergy warning "May contain nuts"!!) – this is a Low HI Food. If you can get the nut in its shell, then buy that instead, as it is the best form of Low HI Food.

This is now where we get onto a couple of questions:

- Which is your favourite part of a supermarket?
- What is the difference between organic food and the rest?
- Is frozen or fresh best?
- Cooked or raw?

The answer to the first question is easy. My favourite part of the supermarket always USED to be the last two aisles – alcohol - because to me this represented relaxation and fun. The rest of the supermarket was just a bunch of food stuffs, most of which was packaged and would be given to me to eat. Or I would use them to make myself food to eat, in saying make myself I mean remove from the freezer, remove from the package and then microwave or place in the oven to cook as it defrosts. NOW? Well now, my favourite part of any supermarket or convenience store is the first bit that you encounter – the MOST colourful part of the store, the fruit and vegetable section, and the rest is just for finding specific additional ingredients so that I may process the raw foods myself into tasty and nutritious meals. Why do I like it so much? It's the vibrant colours and the smells that you get, not only is it visually exciting, but it's a tactile experience too – you get to touch and squeeze the produce, and choose for yourself whether it is fresh or ripe, whether it is going to last or not, you get to choose which one is going to (in your opinion) taste the best. It's a great overall experience!

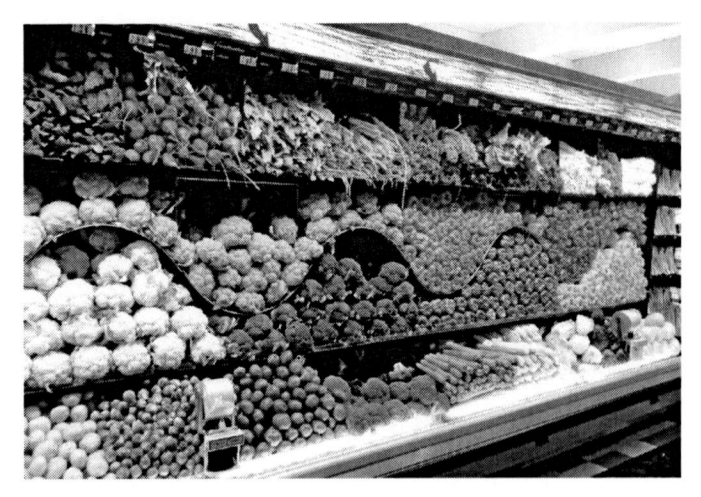

Just look at that, and that's only part of it!

What is the difference between organic and the rest? Organic foods are foods produced by organic farming, which has been operating for almost 100 years, since The Green Revolution of the 1940's. While the standards differ worldwide, organic farming in general features cultural, biological and mechanical practices that foster cycling of resources, promote ecological balance, and conserve biodiversity.

Synthetic pesticides and chemical fertilizers are not allowed, although certain organic pesticides may be used under limited conditions. In general, organic foods are also not processed.

The rest use factory processing techniques and "industrial" agricultural processes. These include the use of chemical pesticides, growth hormones to make the produce bigger and (in the case of meats) leaner; genetic modification which again makes produce bigger, leaner, a certain shape and a richer colour and which lasts longer when on supermarket shelves. The produce is then soaked in preservatives, so that it can complete the journey from source to supermarket (which can take as long as 2 or 3 weeks) and still look fresh. Organic produce is generally sourced more locally, but if not, it can also be subject to the preservative and journey times – so it is good to check the packet when you buy. The journey time means that when fruit and vegetables are picked to go to supermarkets, they are picked at an under ripe stage and ripen to an extent on the journey. Organic foods are expensive, but are slowly becoming more affordable. If you cannot afford to eat organically and want to remove the pesticides and fungicides and other preservatives used on non-organic produce, then you can do this by soaking it in an apple cyder vinegar solution before cooking it.

This brings us to our next question: Is frozen or fresh best? If by "fresh" you mean that you have just pulled it from the ground or tree yourself . . . .THAT is best! If not, then read on.

When food is picked to be frozen, it is picked at its fullest and ripest, but is sadly rarely organically produced. When it is picked, it is full of antioxidants, vitamins, minerals and phytonutrients – the produce is then frozen in this state. The freezing does not destroy all of this goodness, but instead LOCKS it in. The common thing that we then do though is to overcook the produce by microwaving it or boiling it for too long – the best thing to do to heat it through is to steam it.

So, is this produce best cooked or raw? The honest answer is that it depends on the produce. Some fruit and vegetables are best left in their natural state, others are best cooked. For example, tomatoes contain lycopene, a powerful antioxidant that also gives the tomato its red colour, which can be used to improve heart disease and some cancers. Lycopene in its raw form is difficult for the body to use, when cooked, however, the body finds it easier to use the lycopene that it is consuming and therefore tomatoes are better if they are cooked (over-cooking, however, can destroy it). What I do personally is eat produce raw at times and cooked at other times – I allow the situation and meal type to dictate. I may take my produce raw in a juice for example. Whenever I cook though, I only part cook, so that the produce is "al dente" and still quite firm when eaten – I prefer my foods cooked this way and know that it still contains a lot of the goodness that it had in its raw state, at the same time as releasing anything inside that requires a little heat to make it easier to use. Steaming or part boiling is the best way to do this. I rarely fry foods, as frying (especially deep frying) releases free radicals.

FREE RADICALS are unstable molecules missing an electron – these guys are the molecules that cause disease as they oxidise our cells. When we get an imbalance of free radicals, our bodies become imbalanced, and that is when we begin to see symptoms, therefore if we do not balance them out, our bodies continue to develop symptoms. Free radicals are confused and do not know what sort of cell they are supposed to be and become fat cells or tumorous cells or something else. If we expose ourselves to free radicals continually (for example smoking or continually eating fast/fried foods), then they can change and damage the DNA in our cells. If they are allowed to damage the DNA in the cells in our reproductive organs (i.e. sperm and ova), then our ailments and even bad habits/addictions can be passed on to our children, and even to our grandchildren.

ANTIOXIDANTS are the key to balancing, because antioxidants prevent the oxidation process by donating an electron to the free radical and neutralising it! Some antioxidants even bind to certain free radicals and escort them from our body via our waste process. Antioxidants are also useful in boosting our immune system. Our bodies produce antioxidants naturally, but given our modern lifestyles we do not produce sufficient to cope with all of the free radical activity within our bodies – the only way to provide the body with more antioxidants (if you like the weapons to fight the things that attack our cells and make us ill) is to consume them. The greatest source of antioxidants is FRESH WHOLE FOODS.

It is worth also adding that over-exercise or exercising hard but infrequently can cause as much damage as over-eating. This is because when we exercise, the body produces its own free radicals, and the harder we exercise, the more free radicals are produced. If we exercise moderately, 3-5 times a week at regular intervals, then our bodies become used to that and begin to recognise when we are exercising. The body then compensates for the extra free radical activity, by producing greater numbers of antioxidants to neutralise them – so it adjusts its antioxidant content to allow us to exercise safely. If we exercise in big bursts infrequently – for example if we do not exercise all week, but then exercise A LOT at the weekend (maybe we do a fitness class, and a bike ride and a run, and go to the gym too) – then our body does not realise what is happening and therefore cannot compensate by producing more antioxidants, and we are back with the imbalance and symptom scenario.

There is one simple answer to all of these problems – EAT MORE PLANTS! And limit your C.R.A.P. intake: **C**arbonated Drinks – it is believed that one of the main causes of today's obesity epidemic is the overconsumption of soda, soft drinks and processed fruit juices.

Refined Sugar – including flour, sugar, high fructose corn syrup – these are often found in pastries, cakes, cookies, yoghurt and cereals

Artificial colours & flavourings *AND* **A**lcohol – often included in confectionary products, (sweets/candy), soda, soft drinks, crisps or chips. Alcohol is considered a toxin

Processed Products – heavily processed foods such as ice cream, party foods, sausages, ham, smoked and cured meats are all likely to contain refined foods and artificial colours and flavours, as well as trans fats, which are considered a danger to health.

One final thing, before we get into tables to help you choose the right foods. HYDRATION … What do we drink? I've told you in this book so far – don't drink pop or soda, don't drink cordial, don't drink coffee, don't drink dairy milk etc., so what on earth is left ?

Well there are three things left, that are great drinks and do not cause your body problems:

Water – more versatile than it sounds. A lot of people say that they do not like the taste of water. Water should not have a taste, although tap water often does because of the chemicals added to it to purify it and because of the metal pipes we use to get it to our homes. It is best to purchase natural still spring water and even better if you can get it in a glass bottle. If you must use tap water filter it before you use it. Not only does this stop your kettle from furring up, but it will also stop your body from doing so and taste nicer too.

You can drink warm water, as it helps the body to use it more efficiently – when you drink chilled water, the body has to bring it up to body temperature before it can begin to get the best from it. If you drink warm water, then you can put a slice of lemon and a slice of fresh ginger root (peeled) in it. This is great, as both are great for digestion – by drinking a mug of this in a morning instead of a mug of coffee, you are setting your body up to receive food and indigestion will become a thing of the past (so long as this is not the

ONLY step you follow, of course!) It's almost a tea, without tea leaves! This brings us on to the next drink.

Drink TEA – green tea is rich in antioxidants and amongst other things, it has been proven to help prevent cancer. Green tea isn't everyone's cup of tea, so to speak, as it has a bit of an acquired flavour. In order to make it easier to stomach, you can add a teaspoon of local honey. Not only will this sweeten the tea, but it will also make it taste better – one of the side effects of adding local honey to your tea is that it will stop you suffering from hay fever and possibly other allergies. Another option is fruit teas available from your local supermarket – Pukka are best, as they are organically produced and taste GREAT; also companies like Whittards produce "tealess teas" using fruits – they do a beautiful goji berry and acai tealess tea, which you can make in a cafetiere by putting a few spoons of the tea in and then pouring on hot water and leaving to infuse for 5-10 minutes. Tastes great!

Finally JUICE – juicing is NOT a fad; it's more a great way of getting essential nutrients in your body without having to eat the foods that most people these days can't stomach – FRUIT & VEG!! By juicing, you are drinking all of those vitamins, minerals, antioxidants and phytonutrients that you have not been eating.

Juicing does not allow you to eat whatever you like, mindlessly, and get away with it, but is rather part of a healthy lifestyle. We talk about this later in Chapter Eight.

Now move onto the next page and give yourself the Antioxidant Capacity Test (Courtesy The Health Sciences Academy)

ANTIOXIDANT CAPACITY TEST

As we have already discussed, our ability to stay free of disease depends on the balance between our exposure to harmful free radicals and our intake of protective antioxidants.

The antioxidant capacity test [Source: The Health Sciences Academy], allows you to test how well protected your body is, and consists of 3 separate health checks. As you go through each health check, score 1 point for each "yes" answer. Then write your total score for each health check on a piece of paper:

- Symptom Check
- Toxicity Check
- Diet Check

Complete it, work out your total score, and follow the recommendations for your score.

1 - Symptom Check

Score 1 point for each "yes" answer, and then write your total score above:

- Do you frequently suffer from infections (coughs, colds)?
- Do you find it hard to shift an infection?
- Do you have a recurrent infection (cystitis, thrush, earache, herpes, etc.)?
- Do you bruise easily?
- Have you ever suffered from cancer, heart disease, cataracts, diabetes, hypertension, infertility, AMD, measles, mental illness, gingivitis, arthritis?

- Have your parents collectively suffered from two or more of these conditions?
- Do you easily get exhausted after physical exertion?
- Does your skin take a long time to heal?
- Do you suffer from acne, dry skin, or excessive wrinkles for your age?
- Are you overweight?

2 – Toxicity Check

Score 1 point for each "yes" answer, and then write your total score above:

- Do you work or live in a polluted city or by a busy road?
- Do you spend more than two hours in traffic each day?
- Do you spend time in a smoky atmosphere most days?
- Are you quite often exposed to strong sunlight?
- Do you consider yourself unfit?
- Do you exercise excessively?

- Have you smoked for more than five years of your life, less than five years ago?
- Do you smoke now?
- Do you smoke more than ten cigarettes a day?
- Do you have an alcoholic drink each day?

3 – Diet Check

Score 1 point for each "yes" answer, and then write your total score above:

- Do you eat fried food most days?
- Do you eat less than a serving of raw or fresh vegetables each day?
- Do you eat fewer than two pieces of fresh fruit a day?
- Do you rarely eat beans, lentils, quinoa, nuts, seeds, or whole-grains'?
- Do you eat smoked or barbecued food or grill cheese on your food?
- Do you rarely eat foods rich in vitamin C, such as bell peppers, broccoli, cauliflower, cabbage, watercress, lemons, oranges, kiwi, and strawberries?

- Do you rarely eat foods rich in vitamin E, such as tuna, sardines, salmon, beans, peas, sesame seeds, wheat germ, sunflower seeds, and vegetable oils?
- Do you rarely eat foods rich in vitamin A or beta-carotene, such as carrots, squash, pumpkin, cabbage, watercress, sweet potatoes, melon, mangoes, tomatoes, broccoli, beef liver, veal liver?

Now add up your three scores to get a total, and see how you did:

0-10 This is an ideal score, indicating that your health, diet, and lifestyle are consistent with a high level of antioxidant protection. Well done and keep up the great work!

11-15 This is a reasonable score but not ideal. You could increase your power of prevention by increasing your levels of antioxidant protection. Incorporate the recommended antioxidants in your diet (via natural foods or supplements) and follow the Boost Your Antioxidant Protection strategies included in this chapter.

16-20 This is a poor score, indicating plenty of room for improvement. Follow the recommendations from the 11-15 score above. Upgrade your diet with the recommendations contained in this chapter and look at how you can make positive lifestyle changes for increased antioxidant protection.

20+ This is a bad score, putting you in the high-risk group for rapid ageing. You require an antioxidant-rich diet plan. Follow the advice contained in this chapter. You will need to make immediate changes to your diet and lifestyle, plus supplementing antioxidants, to slow down the ageing process and decrease your risk of disease

Tips for boosting your power of prevention, via antioxidants and phytonutrients:

• Eat lots of fresh fruit, especially berries.
• Eat lots of vegetables, especially tender-stem (i.e. Broccoli), spinach, avocado, sweet potatoes, carrots, peas, watercress and broccoli.
• Take a multivitamin and/or a good antioxidant supplement daily.

- Try to avoid pollution, roads with busy traffic, smoky places, direct exposure to strong sunlight, and burned or fried foods.
- Don't over-exercise.

Recommended Antioxidants

Taken either via natural foods (covered in this book) or via antioxidant formulas or capsules, emphasise the following nutrients:

[WARNING: Do NOT take any of these in isolation, rather a combination of them – as we are all different, it is wise to consult a qualified nutritional therapist before taking supplementary formulas or capsules]

- Vitamin A – sweet potatoes, carrots, leafy greens
- Beta-carotene – do not take this on its own, if you smoke. This is found in red, yellow and orange vegetables and fruits

- Vitamin E - found in 'seed' foods, including nuts, seeds and their oils, and vegetables like peas, broad beans, corn and whole grains
- Vitamin C – found in most RAW fruits and vegetables – cooking destroys the Vitamin C contained within
- Zinc – Seafood, beef lamb, wheat germ, spinach, pumpkin seeds, cashews
- Selenium – brazil nuts, tuna, whole wheat, sunflower seeds, pork
- Glutathione – garlic, parsley, onions, cruciferous vegetables
- Cysteine - pork, poultry, eggs, dairy, red peppers, garlic, onions, broccoli, Brussels sprout, oats, granola, wheat germ, sprouted lentils
- Plant-based antioxidants (such as bilberry or pyenogenol)
- Lipoic acid - Foods said to be higher in lipoic acid are liver, spinach, broccoli, Brussels sprouts, and yeast.
- Co-enzyme Q10 - found in meat, fish, nuts, and seeds, it is a vital antioxidant helping to

protect cells from carcinogens and also helping to recycle vitamin E.

The Top 15 MOST Powerful Antioxidant Foods

1. Prunes
2. Raisins
3. Blueberries
4. Blackberries
5. Kale
6. Strawberries
7. Spinach, raw
8. Raspberries
9. Tender-stem (Brocolini)
10. Plums
11. Alfalfa sprouts
12. Spinach, steamed
13. Broccoli
14. Beets
15. Avocado

I hope that some of this information has proved helpful to start you on your journey to a healthier, happier you – as you start to eat better food, those little niggly ailments that annoy and frustrate you because they are always there will begin to disappear. This in turn will make you happier and make you feel better than ever before. The little lifestyle changes like this, or rather adjustments, are the things that will make the biggest differences. Just remember to give yourself time, nothing great ever happened overnight!!

Here is an affirmation that I use every day that keeps me on the straight and narrow, in terms of eating healthy food, because it is true. You need to love yourself before you can expect anyone else to love you.

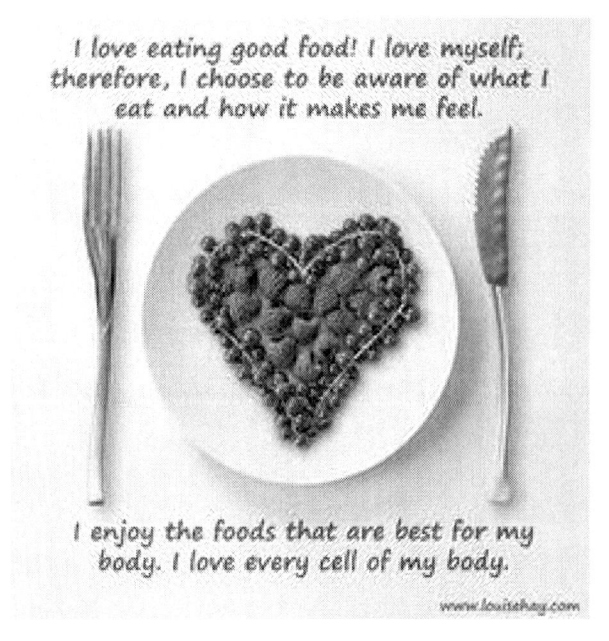

I love eating good food! I love myself; therefore, I choose to be aware of what I eat and how it makes me feel.

I enjoy the foods that are best for my body. I love every cell of my body.

www.louisehay.com

CHAPTER 5 – A Question Of Taste

Something I am often asked about is "taste". A change of diet, a change of lifestyle - "But I love the flavour of chocolate," "I love coffee it tastes so good," "Coffee wakes me up in a morning," "Smoking helps my stress levels," "Alcohol helps me calm down after work," "But fresh bread just smells and tastes so yummy, especially with butter on it," etc. - all of these and more, not only do I hear them from those I help, but. . . . . I used to say the exact same things myself!

Flavour is an amazing thing, and your tongue is an amazing organ! It has thousands of nerve cells on it, which we call taste buds and these send signals to the brain telling it what we are eating, and we react to different flavours in different ways. Food manufacturers exploit this by filling foods with flavours that they know our brains will love. They also assail our noses and sense of smell – ever wondered why the moment that you step into a supermarket you can smell bread? They PUMP the smell into the air conditioning system, even when they are not cooking – they use an artificial scent!!

8 months ago, I used to smoke 20 a day, eat chocolate, live on a staple diet of cheese rolls, burgers and biscuits or cookies, drink wine and beer EVERY night and drink about 6 cups of coffee a day MINIMUM. Now, I no longer smoke, I no longer drink coffee, I do not eat bread, or dairy, and my dependence on sugary snacks like biscuits and cakes has gone. I rarely eat chocolate, and on the occasions that I do, I only eat raw organic plain chocolate, my diet is a balanced and nutritional vegetarian fare and I drink in moderation, mindfully. In short I have not only completely turned my life around, but I have also turned my health around!! So I speak from experience.

Every so often, your body regenerates - it replaces every cell when it dies (and each cell has its own life span) with a good cell. It's a known fact that 95% of all disease suffered by humans is related to their environment - what we eat, what we drink, what we breathe, what we do and what we think. Your diet (whether good or bad) tells your body which genes to turn on and off, and your body acts accordingly. Stands to reason then that if you put negative into your body, then you will get a negative body. . . .Put positives in, and the results will speak for themselves.

So what happened that made me change my life? I didn't have a heart attack or any major disease, although I have suffered previously from two heart attacks, I had a life event. This negative life event (a marriage ended) caused me to hit the cigarettes and booze harder than ever, and to hide myself away. One day I woke up and realised that the effects of my Parkinson's Disease were getting worse and so I had to go and visit my doctor as I was finding it difficult to function - I put little faith in the medical profession, believing that they are in arms with the pharmaceutical companies and only want me for my pill popping abilities! I visited and got my tablets (which I am now off - a SIDE EFFECT of leading a healthy lifestyle!!), but also got checked for vitals whilst there - my blood pressure was elevated to a dangerous level, my cholesterol was higher than it should be etc. etc. - and my doctor told me that I was headed for my third heart attack, but that this would be my last. . . . Basically it would be massive and I would die.

About a week later, with the doctor's words ringing around my head, I got into my car, took a cigarette from the pack and lit it - it was the last one in its pack . . . this was on July 4th 2014 and I said to myself there and then - right this is it, no more, and I stopped. This was the start of my lifestyle change. Stop smoking and, immediately, smell and taste explode and these senses are heightened, as they have been dulled by the nicotine. The sensations are endless - everything tastes SO MUCH better. Well this spurred me on, and I started going to exercise classes (I've always kept fit - the last few years at home on my own), as I wanted to repair my lungs and make them work properly. I met a nutritionist who introduced me to organic food - her name was Gilly-Marie Harvey and we are working together to help people change their lives. She also explained in great detail what the processed foods I had been eating were doing to my body - OMG I never even realised what they put in that stuff - much of it poison, much of it carcinogenic, much of it fat-producing and much of it ADDICTIVE! It was definitely time to change.

Then in August, I met the love of my life. A woman I had first met 20+ years ago, and then fallen in love with about 15 years ago, when unfortunately we were both in other relationships. She was a vegetarian - something I had wanted to do for a few years - and subscribed to the same opinions and ideals as Gilly. My diet changed from that moment, and I cut meat out of my diet. Now this is not for everyone, and you can eat meat and be healthy, for me though it was about my ideals with regard to animals, as well as my health. Organic Guinea Pig (my lifestyle analysis and nutritional therapy business) had been in operation for a while and I had been trying different foods and experimenting, but now change was upon me.

My new partner would bring bags of food in from shopping - taking out asparagus and fennel and chicory and all types of things that I had heard of, but never tried. She would smile, brandishing an avocado, and I would look at it, pull a face and say "Don't like those" just like a petulant teenager. She was patient and would ask "Have you ever tried one" and I would look at my feet shaking my head! It was amusing when I look back. . . what options did I have though, other than to try them? So that is what I did, and I found that I appreciated these new flavours and textures that I was being introduced to - my mouth was flooded with these rich delightful experiences, and showed it's appreciation by flooding my mouth with saliva and sending positive messages to my brain.

I then stopped drinking coffee completely - something else that dulled my taste buds. But what did I have instead? I started to drink hot water with a slice of lemon and a slice of ginger in - not only does this taste refreshingly bright and clean, but it wakes you up and sets up your body to receive food. Amazing - and it tastes so beautiful, after my first mouthful I felt healthier. The zinginess of the lemon and strength of the ginger combine to leave you feeling clean inside. To de-stress, I eat or juice an orange - Vitamin C is an awesome stress reduction tool and much better for you than cigarettes and alcohol.

When you choose to change your lifestyle, you choose to give your taste buds the gift of life!! It's a gradual thing and won't happen overnight, but if you stick with it, you will change yourself for life. Like any bad habit - it's quicker and easier to grab a burger or a sandwich - it has to be changed for a good habit - you will learn techniques that mean you CAN get yourself a healthy meal every night. Being healthy does not have to be boring, and we shall share some of our recipes at the end of the book, so that you can indulge without the guilt, and if you do indulge, as we all do at those special times (such as Christmas), then you can counteract that indulgence by being strictly healthy for a few weeks. If you indulge for a day (say your birthday), then so long as you are eating healthy before and after that day, then it's OK and there is no need to feel guilty (this is Freedom Mentality)

So is it a question of taste? No, it's a question of adaptation and being a little more adventurous with foods. As well as retraining your body to accept nutrients and antioxidants, and allowing it to feel and work better, you have to retrain your mind. Taste is all in the mind, we have our minds programmed by the food and drink manufacturers, who tell us what smells and tastes good, and we go out and buy it, we put it in our body, and eventually our body goes out of balance and gets sick. Your mind will LOVE learning how all of the wonderful flavours of nature taste. YOU have the POWER to choose, and the POWER to change - use it. Other SIDE EFFECTS of a natural organic lifestyle include:

Increased libido – many of the foods you will be eating improve the body's blood flow and therefore you will feel recharged and you will feel happier and more positive.

Increased energy – a lot of the processed foods that we have come to rely on, not just junk, but also tinned soups and microwave meals (we won't get on to microwaves!) contain ingredients that slow us down and make us feel low and lacking in energy. By removing these from our diets, and eating natural whole foods filling ourselves with wonderful phytonutrients, we become more energised. I for one have discovered this as I have changed my lifestyle.

Better cleaner brighter skin – many of the antioxidants that you will be eating promote clean and healthy skin. In addition to improving any skin conditions that you may have, eating a proper whole, nutrition-filled diet will also CLEAR your wrinkles! Something else I have noticed – so many friends who have seen me recently have told me how much better and younger I look.

Less reliance on prescribed medication – when we eat or drink processed foods especially those with lots of refined sugar in, the processed sugar gives us a very quick "happy spike", but that then dies away quickly and we get a sudden low. When we get a lot of these, we feel unhappy and it has been shown to lead to depression in people. When we feel low a lot, and seem unable to explain it, we go to the doctor. The doctor will then diagnose it as depression and will prescribe tablets, many of which are also addictive. We then go back every month for more tablets, and end up reliant on them.

When you change your diet, you really do change everything – because you are no longer putting these foods into your body, the spikes and lows no longer occur, because the sugar in fruit and vegetables is released more slowly than refined sugars, and over a period of time, therefore you get more of a gentle wave of happiness. I cannot remember the last time that I felt down, despite many bad things happening, and I put this down to nutrition – I am always on the up! Since starting to eat whole foods with proper nutritional value, not only have I been happier, but I have also stopped taking the prescription meds that I was reliant on for blood pressure and Parkinson's Disease – all with the consent of a medical professional of course.

And there are also more benefits:

How we react to taste, and our personal tastes in food can be reprogrammed, we just have to have the passion to improve our lives (something you obviously have, as you are reading this book, and got this far!) and the persistence to keep trying . . .oh, and the willpower to stop putting that C.R.A.P. (that we are programmed to believe tastes so good) into our baskets and trolleys, and ultimately our mouths.

Take the test, and answer the question for yourself!!

> "THE FOOD YOU EAT CAN BE EITHER THE SAFEST & MOST POWERFUL FORM OF MEDICINE or THE SLOWEST FORM OF POISON."
>
> Ann Wigmore

CHAPTER SIX – The Role Of Exercise

Exercise plays a very important part in our health and wellbeing. Whether it is leading an active lifestyle, whether it is going to the gym, or it may even be a mixture of the two. Either way, it pays to be active – lead a sedentary lifestyle and life will catch up with you at some point.

An active lifestyle gets you out and about – you can become a member of a rambling club, it's not just old people that do it you know, and if in your area it is, then why not start up a rambling club of your own with a few friends. Rambling gets you out and about in the fresh air, and more importantly in the countryside and in nature, where the air is less toxic and improves the body's environment. Just leading an active life – movement – is so important to the body's health and means that you are keeping all of your organs working and giving them the opportunity to work.

If you think of your body like a car – if you lead a sedentary lifestyle, that is like leaving your car on the drive and only starting it once a month, just to make sure it's still there if you need it (maybe when you go shopping) ; if you lead an active lifestyle, that means that you are starting your car every day, taking it off the drive and for a little trip or run round somewhere – this keeps all of the cogs and parts oiled and lubricated and the engine (the body's organs) is kept in tip top shape! It's not about the body work so much, it's about the engine, and making sure it's working at its best. You can also involve nutrition in this analogy – you would not use cooking oil in your car's engine to lubricate it, you make sure you use the right stuff and the best that you can afford to put in. If you put junk in your car and then try and drive it, it's going to break pretty quickly. *Your body is no different to your car!* Strange to think, that a lot of us think more about our car than we do our own body, huh?

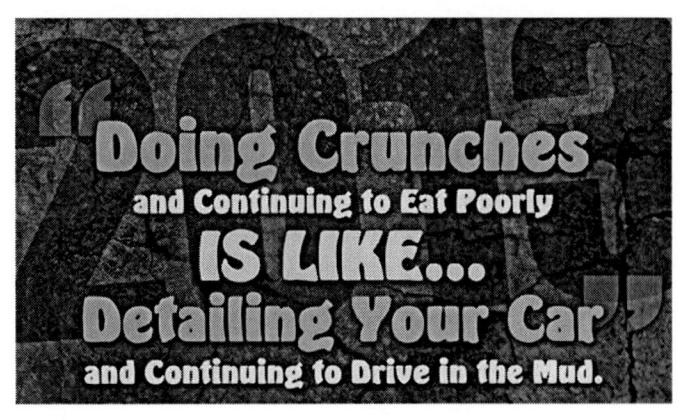

> **"Doing Crunches and Continuing to Eat Poorly IS LIKE... Detailing Your Car and Continuing to Drive in the Mud.**

Going to the gym gives us more options to get the inside AND the outside in shape. Too much credence is put on body size and shape, weight, muscle definition. The thing is that somebody may have an absolutely perfectly toned and muscularly defined body, but their organs may be shot, their cells may be damaged. It's great to look good on the outside, but if you do not pay as much attention to the inside, then you can still get sick. We've all heard about the guys who were in perfect shape, but dropped down from a heart attack in the middle of some form of exercise right?

Well, that is because although they trained hard, they did not fuel that training with the right food – looked after the outside but not the inside.

Many people will go to the gym and lift weights, but do no cardio vascular exercise – in essence their definition will be spot on, their single lift strength will be amazing, but their cardio vascular resilience will be zero! You cannot do one without the other; in fact you can do neither successfully without the correct nutrition.

Gyms and sports centres offer all sorts of services – swimming, gymnasiums, classes, badminton, tennis and more at times. Swimming is great exercise, especially when you are just starting to exercise (with correct nutrition and doctor's permission of course) and is also good for toning, some places will also offer Aqua Aerobics, which is brilliant to start – it uses the resistance of the water.

Gyms are great, but can be intimidating for many. Lots of people go to gyms in groups of two or more, and they are also a great place for "Peacocks" as I call them. "Peacocks" are people who strut around the equipment, watching themselves in the mirror – their technique is out, but they love to watch their muscles under stress – and looking around to see who is watching their amazing ability on the equipment. These are not the guys to watch or follow – they will whack on the weight but their technique will be completely incorrect. These guys stand more chance of injury than they do of developing a healthy and truly fit body. Muscle definition and bulk does not equal fit and healthy.

Badminton, tennis, squash is all great all over body workouts – they get the heart rate up and employ pretty much every muscle in your body. The only problem with these three activities is the fact that it takes two to tango – you need a partner to play with. Maybe you can play with a friend or your partner.

There are all sorts of fitness classes, the most popular being – Spin, Body Pump, Body Combat, Aerobics, Yoga and Zumba. Most of these lift the heart rate and tone the muscles; they do not build muscle bulk. They are all great all-over body workouts – yes even Yoga is an all-over body workout. Classes are great and combined with an active lifestyle, at two or three classes a week can really help you to maintain a healthy inside and good looking outside! Taking two or three classes a week, and leading a sedentary lifestyle the rest of the time, at the same time as eating incorrectly, can actually do more harm than good, and you will not see the same positive results. I will explain this later on in this chapter.

Boot Camps are also becoming a very popular phenomenon, and seem to be springing up pretty much everywhere all over the western world. I love boot camp and I do several each week, but I also lead a very active lifestyle, at the same time as eating mindfully and getting my nutrition right. Since starting regular boot camp, I have lost weight in the form of the fatty areas of my body. Mainly my stomach and my hips – you know those things we call "love handles"? Well I have renamed them – I refer to them as "Complacency Inhibitors". Whilst I can still see them in the mirror, I cannot become complacent about my nutritional intake, or about my exercise. I will not become complacent about my lifestyle balance!

Boot camps (so long as the personal trainer who is giving the training knows his stuff) give a good mix of cardio vascular work and toning exercises – again they are not designed to build bulk and muscle, they are designed to help you lose fat and tone your body. You cannot exercise whilst continuing to eat junk food and cakes, and expect a healthy body – the balance needs to be right. The thing that I like most about boot camps is that there are no "Peacocks" at boot camp, there is no intimidation – everybody is there for the same purpose and to do the same exercises for the same reason. There is a certain amount of friendly rivalry, a great atmosphere and a really positive attitude within the group. You help each other, you motivate each other, and you form good bonds, helping each other to reach your individual goals – between all shapes and sizes, all levels of ability, and all ages.

So how much is too much exercise? Where should we start? I am too big to exercise, how much weight do I need to lose before I can start to exercise? Everyone has an opinion. If you have not exercised before, or you are not used to exercise; if you are overweight or suffer from chronic illnesses, ALWAYS consult your doctor before starting an exercise (or diet) program.

Too much exercise will make you sick. If you are not used to exercise, you may feel sick, experience chest pains, find it difficult to breathe etc. The trick is to listen to your body, and when your body feels like it's telling you to slow down or stop, then answer it by doing just that – DO NOT push yourself too hard. If you are heavily overweight or suffer from chronic illness, then it would be best to start slowly and build up as you begin to feel more comfortable with exercise – don't just jump into Boot Camp. A starting point would be a walk – 5 minutes down the road and then 5 minutes back. Once your body has got used to this, it can be extended to 10 minutes and so on, until you are walking for 60 minutes plus a day. If you then want to start running, gently, then that is fine, but again, it should be run for 5 minutes and then walk for 10, and repeat. Again build it up from 5 minutes, until you are running for 60 minutes.

When you get to the point of walking for an hour every day without any adverse effects, then you may want to visit a gym and start building your muscles to a normal level and then toning your body, or you may wish to start at a boot camp. Both of these options will give you a good start – a good gym or boot camp will assess your level of ability and fitness before allowing you to embark on an exercise program. They will ask questions about health conditions and about lifestyle in order to ascertain your level of ability and fitness, and many will do a fitness test, where they take measurements and take a look at your start point. The fitness test is great, because then every month or so you can have another to measure your progress.

If you elect to go straight into exercise classes, you will get none of these, and will be expected in most cases to perform at the same level of ability as every other member of the class – a lot are also choreographed to music, and therefore there are rhythms and moves to learn too. If you wish to start exercise classes, the best idea would be to ask for advice from a member of the fitness team as to which classes would best suit you – be honest in your explanation of where you are, you will not be judged or laughed at, and you will then get the best advice and ultimately results.

The best exercise is MODERATE exercise – which means do not have a massive exercise blast once or twice a week, rather have several medium "blasts" at regular intervals. It is not a brilliant idea to exercise each and every day of the week (in which I mean go to the gym, or workout – it's fine to walk every day, but not do a 10k run every day!), as when you workout, your muscles tear and rip, or they are pushed close to max capacity. So you need to take rest days in-between your workout days to allow your muscles to repair.

MODERATE also means that we do not workout for prolonged periods of time, 45 minutes to an hour 3 or 4 times a week is sufficient. During a workout you are really pushing your muscles and your internal organs (heart and lungs) to capacity and it is extremely important that we do not push them to capacity for too long.

Stretching is also an important part in the role of exercise. Stretching keeps your body and limbs supple, as when you exercise your muscles and tendons shorten and you then stretch afterwards in order to lengthen them back out and "relax" them. I cannot emphasise the importance of stretching enough – failure to stretch after exercise (including initially walking) will have lasting negative effects on your body and you will eventually lose flexibility and range of movement in your limbs. If you wish to take stretching and relaxation a little further, then YOGA could be for you. Yoga is an amazing exercise, which is holistically healing, positive, relaxing and exceptionally good for body and mind. During a yoga class, you will meditate and experience deep relaxation. At the same time, you will learn stretching exercises that will help your limbs to become more flexible. In the same way that in the gym the weights you lift will become heavier, the flexibility in your limbs will increase from little flexibility to great flexibility. Due to stretching correctly after exercise and practicing yoga occasionally, I am now able to touch my toes, and get my body into all sorts of positions that I was not able to achieve before.

If money is a problem, and gyms and the like are beyond financial reach, or you do not have the confidence to go to these places, and then do not despair. You can still exercise, but do it at home – be sure to do your research from reliable sources with regard to exercises and technique, and include both cardio vascular and muscular exercises. There is no need to buy expensive equipment. A couple of 1 or 2 litre bottles of water will suffice as weights, your stairs will make a great place for cardio vascular exercise – you can use the entire staircase or just step up and down using one step. You can walk, you can run, you can cycle in order to get the heart rate up. There are also other exercises such as burpies, mountain climbers, jumping jacks etc. Using your bottles of water (these can also be filled with sand if you so desire) you can then do bicep curls and other upper body exercises. Tricep dips can be done off a dining room chair or stair or sofa or coffee table. The leg muscles can be toned by doing squats, lunges and the like, and the stomach muscles by doing sit ups! All of this at zero or at least very little cost!

So where does nutrition fit into this? And why can too much exercise be bad for you? Some things you may have heard of before are *free radicals* and *antioxidants.* So let me explain what they are, how they relate to each other, and how exercise affects how they work.

Free Radicals

Free radicals are unstable molecules, missing an electron, making them unstable. If left unchecked they can cause damage to living cells and DNA (and hence cause disease and also can change genetic markers thus passing the disease down through generations through reproduction (if they affect the reproductive organs and cells)). Free radicals are thought to be a by-product from a number of causes including environmental factors, unhealthy food, smoking, radiation and a number of other sources.

Antioxidants

Antioxidants are chemical compounds that are able to quench the effects of free radicals by donating one of their spare electrons and neutralising the free radical. Scientists have now identified a number of these antioxidants. Most are naturally occurring plant compounds.

If an imbalance of free radicals to antioxidants occurs, and there are more free radicals than there are antioxidants, these unstable molecules travel around the body and get their missing electrons from other cells that cannot afford to donate one. By doing this, they damage the cells, affecting the cell DNA and causing the cells to mutate. This is when symptoms begin to show and we begin to get ill. Depending on the type of cell affected and the place in the body, this can cause all sorts of chronic disease such as asthma, heart problems, and cancer.

Where does this fit in with exercise? Well, our bodies produce both free radicals and antioxidants in equal measure, so that we remain in balance. When we exercise however, we produce an excess of free radicals, because we are oxidising our cells. When we exercise too hard, or have infrequent bursts of heavy exercise, we naturally produce many more free radicals, and the body cannot pump out sufficient antioxidants to neutralise them. This means that we suddenly have an imbalance in the body, and the body begins to show symptoms of illness, especially if we keep repeating this behaviour. Because of the irregular exercise and intensity of it, exercising in this manner can do more harm than good.

When we exercise moderately and regularly, however, our bodies get used to the cues and start producing extra antioxidants automatically. This is because the body realises the trigger for us exercising and knows that there are going to be extra free radicals, and so produces more antioxidants to compensate for that. Our body therefore remains in balance.

How does nutrition fit in? By eating the correct foods and getting the nutrition right, we can help the body in its production of antioxidants, to neutralise the free radicals and help it to prevent imbalance and therefore disease – chronic and otherwise. By eating the correct foods, rich in antioxidants we can help our bodies to maintain good health, even to get better.

Foods that help you get the most from your workout, at the same time as helping your body cope with it:

Bananas – slow release carbs – bananas are a great pre workout food. They will help to replace potassium (lost in sweat) and help with energy levels. Bananas also help to reduce the build-up of lactic acid during your workout. They are also good eaten after exercise for the same reason.

Beetroot juice (fresh) – can be diluted with water and drunk whilst working out. Beetroot opens up the blood vessels and allows blood to flow through them more easily, thus making your body work more efficiently. Beets are also rich in vital antioxidants.

Berries – Berries are great providers of antioxidants, to help neutralise all of those free radicals, and assist your body in dealing with them. Blueberries, raspberries, cranberries, blackberries, raisins, prunes and cherries are among the best.

Dark green vegetables – such as kale, spinach, broccoli and sprouts included in a meal before or after a workout help the body in its production of antioxidants, as they are all antioxidant rich foods.

A bowl of porridge made with nut or oat milk and mixed with blueberries and banana can be a great pre or post workout meal.

If you are going to eat a meal (be it porridge, salad or a cooked meal) before a workout then it is advisable to do so at least an hour before hand, which will give the gut the opportunity to begin processing the food that you have provided for it.

"Exercise is King, Nutrition is Queen, Put them together and you have a kingdom" ~ Jack Lalanne (The Godfather of Fitness)

CHAPTER SEVEN – Positive Happiness

"Like a river, I will cut a new path when I meet an obstacle!"

In this chapter I will explain how to have and maintain a healthy and positive mind, and my philosophy on it. At the same time, I will give you my trademarked system on how to treat the negative stuff!

Someone once told me that you never get more than you can deal with – sometimes it feels like you've been dealt bad hand after bad hand, but every one is a lesson to be learned, and once learned you can move on. Some people never learn the lesson that they are being taught and remain in a self-perpetuating cycle for their whole lives. Others are fast learners, or intuitive, or are just in tune with their lives – where this happens, those people are the ones we perceive to be successful! Took me 40 odd years to work this out, but now that I have it, life is a dream!

I have had many lessons sent my way – I have lost everything – including a dream holiday home in Orlando that I visited 2 or 3 times per year - and been down and out with nothing to my name. I have had various other personal tragedies too, but now, using this system, I find it easy to deal with pretty much everything life throws at me. Now, when a lesson is thrown at me, the first question I ask is: "What are you teaching me?" and I focus on solving the puzzle, so that I may move on as quickly as possible.

Sometimes you are being taught a life lesson; Other times you are being pushed in a certain direction; Another lesson is in relationships; Sometimes it's simply a nudge to tell you it is time to move on.

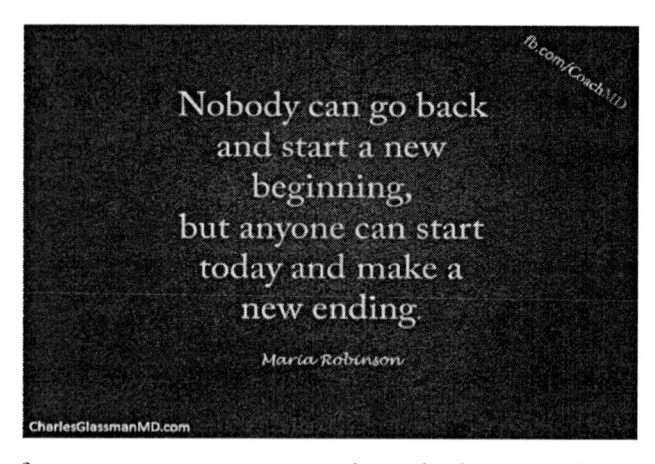

> Nobody can go back and start a new beginning, but anyone can start today and make a new ending.
>
> *Maria Robinson*

Before we move on to my trademarked system, let's consider *"Resistance vs Acceptance"*. These two are very important when it comes to positive thinking. You cannot change what happened yesterday, you cannot predict what will happen tomorrow, and all you can do is shape your today. If you think about it, this makes sense. Many people spend their whole lives worrying about the future or regretting what they didn't do yesterday, instead of accepting that yesterday has passed and that what they do today will shape their futures – this acceptance makes life so much easier to live, decisions easier to make, and negativity easier to cope with.

It can go with almost anything – many of us are frustrated by something that a partner or friend does. So much so that when they do it, we cannot help but comment, or pull them up, in short draw attention to it. We resist their behaviour, because it frustrates us – the comment or reaction is our resistance. Let's look at their behaviour another way.

They are themselves, an individual, a single entity – they may be connected to us spiritually or in some other way, but nothing will ever stop them being themselves. If we accept this simple fact, then we will never have a problem with anything they do, and we will no longer feel that frustration. Everybody is an individual and as such we are all unique, with our own unique way of living – no two people, anywhere in the world, live their lives in exactly the same way. We therefore should reduce our expectations of others to zero – other than the usual manners and courtesy of course. So, if we show acceptance, we can deal with the issue and move on – there is no need to comment, to feel annoyance, to pass judgement or to allow it to frustrate us. We can smile at their little quirk and remember why it is we became their friend or partner in the first place.

Here is another example. Somebody is ill, and they get frustrated by their symptoms. They may shout or scream, or in worst cases get depressed by how their illness makes them feel - resistance. If, instead, we accept that our symptoms are part of the illness and therefore unavoidable – they are a sign that our body is healing itself or displaying discomfort because of what is happening to it. By resisting we make the situation feel 10 times worse – if we can accept what is happening then it is so much easier to deal with, and we begin to feel better.

Easier said than done you say!! Well yes, you are right, but as with every other habit, practice makes perfect. The more we accept, the easier it becomes, the more often we practice acceptance, then the more accepting of things we become. When acceptance becomes part of your everyday life, regardless of the situation you are faced with, then life becomes easier to live.

This is the first thing you need to do in order to have and maintain a healthy and positive mind. Once you have mastered acceptance, it's time to start looking at life in a different way.

Where does happiness come from? To some happiness involves having the best possessions – the biggest house, the fastest, smartest car, the flashiest jewellery, the best designer clothes etc. etc. YAWN!!!! Do possessions really make you truly happy? or are you trying to make up for something that you are lacking? True happiness comes from within, from deep inside your soul. I have no possessions of any value. I know that I could walk out of my front door and leave everything behind without looking back. This would horrify so many people – so, I would take my pets (but I do not class them as possessions, they are sentient beings), but everything else is just a "thing".

Ever since I lost everything 10 years ago, I have never looked at anything the same. I had to find happiness within – prior to this I had everything money could buy, nice, expensive stuff and lots of it. Then I had a motorcycle crash and hit a brick wall – I broke both arms, I could not work my highly paid job, I got fired. The thought of losing my nice car and dream motorcycle (I had two), my original oil painting by a modern surrealist master, my jewellery, watches, everything I prized, was soul destroying. When eventually it went, I realised that I did not miss any of it, not for a single second, in fact life was easier. No longer was I trying to outdo my neighbour, constantly stressed by the fact they had upgraded and I hadn't. I realised that I didn't care anymore – none of that mattered.

People say that this happens because you have nothing, and so you "pay lip" to it. it's not true, however, this happens because you have acceptance for the fact that it had to go, to show you that it did not matter . . . a realisation, one of life's lessons learned.

True happiness happens and increases with each and every one of these realisations, because with each lesson you learn, you grow. Your soul grows, your mind grows and you grow as a person – your brain and mind start to work in a different way and your heart swells with happiness, because you do not need anything but yourself to be happy.

My Trademarked SN System

What is my trademarked SN System? It is a proven system for looking at life and remaining positive, even though life keeps on throwing you curve balls.

SN stands for Sat Nav – in short we can look at life through the screen of a Sat Nav. When we want to take a journey in our car, and more recently with mobile devices, if we are walking somewhere, then we get that black box out and attach it to our windshield. We then take the co-ordinates for our destination and we program them into our Sat Nav. We even have a NAME for our little friend (mine is called Shirley – it's a long story) and some of us talk to them!! The Sat Nav then begins talking back, telling us which way to proceed, until finally we hear "You are now arriving at your destination". Job done – it's easy and simple . . .I remember having to use map books, and boy was that tough!!

My belief is that life is already planned out – we have a start point (birth), and we have a destination, which is death. All of the routes we take in-between are the results of our internal Sat Nav showing us the way. What does "Shirley" do when she gets lost? She reprograms her route. How do we do the same? We make a decision on what to do next and when we make that decision, we are reprograming our internal Sat Nav. We hit a dead end, we reroute.

When many (me included at one time) hit a dead end, or encounter a problem or obstacle, we feel like it is the end of our journey. But, what do successful people do? They keep on moving, sometimes it seems impossible for them to, but they do – they keep on finding ways around the obstacles. As the quote at the start of this chapter stated – Just like the river!

How do we reprogram successfully? How do we know if we have made the right decision? The truth is we don't. If you get really lost on a journey, your Sat Nav will keep on changing the route until you are back on track, and that's exactly what we need to do.

In my life, I have had 4 long term relationships – each time they ended I thought it was the end of the road, but then I reprogrammed my internal Sat Nav. I ended up on a different road and followed it until I got lost again, each time reprogramming. And this is how I look at every problem I encounter:

- Acceptance of the problem
- Realisation of the lesson I am being taught
- Reprogram based on that realisation

The result, my internal happiness increases, and I grow a little more in wisdom and knowledge. I make progress towards realising my next dream – my new destination (me and dreams have a history, I seem to achieve all of my dreams), and once that is reached, I reprogram again. Those who fail to do these three things are the people who get stuck, and remain lost in life – the guys who believe that they were never meant to be successful. They never move forwards with their lives. The truth is . . . we are ALL meant to be successful – the difference between those who are and those who aren't is that those who are dare to BELIEVE.

Those who follow this system move forwards, grow in wisdom, are happy in life, and motivated. More importantly, these are the guys who are the most SUCCESSFUL at what they do – these are the people that we look up to, the people who inspire us. People like Richard Branson, Jason Vale, Joe Cross, Gerry Robert.

Who, like this, inspires you? Take a look at their life story – they will most certainly have ups, but inevitably they will also have had their downs, their problems, their obstacles. Delve deeper and you will find out that each time, they reset their Sat Nav and moved forwards a little further. Be inspired by their story, because if they can do it, then so can you.

Meditation is important. Meditation is about focusing on the now and removing all other thoughts from your mind – clearing your mind completely. This helps you to relax, focus, gain perspective, "reset" your thoughts and more. There are several ways, and you can meditate many times in a day – it's not all hippies sitting around in circles cross-legged with their hands in the air "omming". I do mini meditations through the day – I will stand for a few seconds, clasp my hands in front of me and take 5 deep breaths in through my nose, and let them out through my mouth, remaining mindful of the air going in through my mouth and into my lungs and then returning out of my body. This is just sufficient to calm my mind, slow my heart, and relax me, resetting my thoughts and allowing me to move along from wherever I have got stuck. I also find this technique great in-between sets at boot camp – it helps me recover my heart and lung function more rapidly.

Something I learned recently about meditation was via a children's book! There are a set of children's books about meditation and compassion, which are amazing. This is what we should be teaching our children to do in order to help them to deal with life – I certainly wish I had learned 40 years ago, instead of now! This method can also be used for family mediation as well – 10 minutes a day is all that you need. For this technique, you will need a bell or gong and a snow globe:

1. Bang the bell / gong and shake the snow globe
2. Put the snow globe in front of you and watch it
3. As you watch it, breathe in deeply and be mindful of the air flowing in through your mouth and filling your lungs, and then feel it flowing out

4. Imagine each of the pieces of "snow" flying around in the chaos of the globe, is one of your thoughts, negative emotions, angry thoughts, and watch as they float to the floor and settle there, gone from the chaos
5. Feel your mind clear as you concentrate on the now, and feel your thoughts disappear
6. Once all of the snow has settled and the globe, like your mind, is clear and free from chaos, ring the bell to signal the end of the meditation
7. Keep on being mindful of the stillness and the emptiness of the current moment until the bell has stopped ringing
8. Try not to smile!!!

"True happiness, comes from bringing all your attention to whatever you are doing right now. Today is all around us" ~ Happy Panda. Be in the now, now without thinking about anything else, focus on the now, enjoy the now – this came from a children's book, and Monkey got it.... "mind-full, like your mind is full of the present, full of right now".... There's no room for anything else. Enjoy

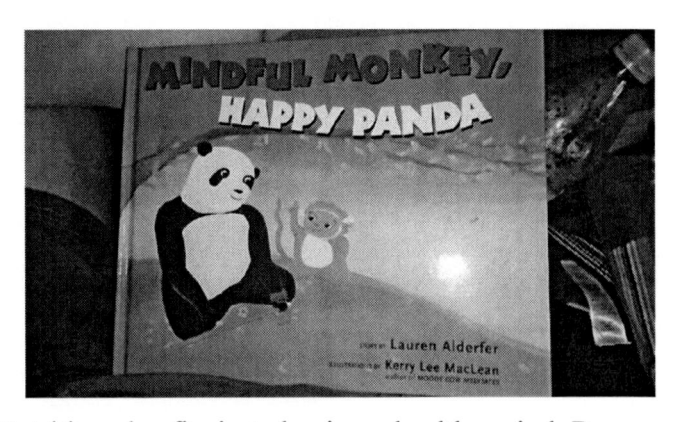

Nutrition also fits in to having a healthy mind. By eating the right foods and drinking in a healthy way, your mind will become the very essence of healthy – in terms of positive thought processes, happiness, and positive energy. Many processed foods, refined salts, flours and sugars, and most carbonated drinks, contain chemical ingredients which when ingested can create very quick elevated chemical "food highs" which are followed by just as quick "food lows", which can lead to depression, anxiety and even over-eating (which of course leads to obesity, low self-esteem etc. etc.) – all of these are negative feelings, leading to negative thought processes. The right foods not only boost the feel good hormones in your brain, but by doing so will also help to boost your self-esteem and confidence. We already know that if we put the right food into our bodies, then we get the right things out of our bodies.

This also fuels your mind. The right food in the right quantities will do wonders for your positive happiness. Combine nutrition with exercise – another positivity booster because of the feelgood hormones released when we exercise and the increased self-esteem we get from looking and feeling better – meditation and a positive way of looking at life, and you have The OGP System (that's my – The Organic Guinea Pig - system for life). Give it a go.

"Don't wait for the perfect moment ; Take the moment, and make it perfect" ~ Zoey Sayward

CHAPTER EIGHT – Juicing As A Refresher

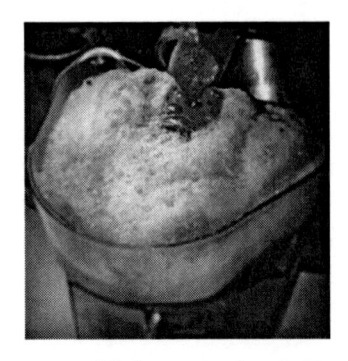

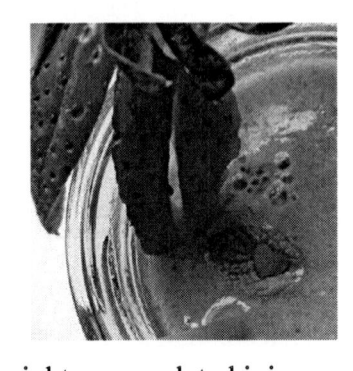

Beautiful aren't they? To the right, a completed juice – specially concocted for Valentine's Day 2015 – we called it "Cupids Arrow". And on the left, this is what it looks like when you are creating a juice, this is the outlet to our Optimum 600 slow juicer. The rainbow colours show that this juice contains many vitamins, minerals and phytonutrients that help the body and mind to be healthy, fit and full of energy. Doesn't it look so much better than the beige blandness of chips and bread and pie or roasted chicken that so many people eat? That is because good food is bright and colourful and fresh.

If you forget what you were told about eating 5 a day, just eat a rainbow!!

So what is "juicing" and how does it work?

Firstly what is juice? Juice is the water which the plants have taken in through the soil, and absorbed. As the water is absorbed, it is absorbed with many nutrients and minerals from the soil which have been dissolved in that water. These micronutrients give the water contained within the fruit and vegetables its vivid colours. This is what we call "Juice" and it is the true nectar of nature, and the ORIGINAL fast food.

Juicing isn't, as many newspapers and media reports have stated, the new diet fad or fashion. Juicing is not about losing weight – the weight loss is a side effect – juicing is about giving your body the essential nutrients it needs, in a format that is easy for it to absorb, so that it can be kick-started into repairing itself from the inside.

When you juice, you remove the insoluble fibre from the fruit, squeezing all of the soluble fibre (in liquid form) from it. The insoluble fibre is discarded, in the form of pulp, and the soluble fibre is the end product. When we eat fruit as it is, we consume both soluble and insoluble fibres, but our body has to spend time digesting the insoluble and extracting the soluble, which is then absorbed into the body, which benefits from all of the nutritional goodness contained within. By extracting the juice, and drinking it, there is no work for the stomach to do in digesting and extracting, and therefore the goodness is absorbed easily and in a quicker time straight into the body and the benefits are felt and seen more quickly.

Many will refer to doing a "5 day juicing detox" or a "7 day juicing detox" or "28 day juicing detox" or anywhere in between. It's not really the correct word "detox", but "kick-start" is. When you juice, you are essentially kick-starting your system into accepting healthy and nutritious foods, vitamins, minerals and phytonutrients by the glassful!

When you do a juice "detox" you eat no solid food, but drink just juice – four a day – for the length of your detox. People like Jason Vale and Joe Cross are the best known "go to" juicers, which the masses are following. I have met them both and seen them both live, and they are amazing people, who openly admit that they use the word "detox" because it conjures the correct mental image in people's minds, and therefore people automatically identify with what they are doing.

The juices you drink ARE NOT those juices that are commercially available in grocery stores, they are made by you FRESH every day from FRESH produce that you have purchased in the grocery store. Fruit AND vegetables – not just one or the other, but both, mixed together in the same glass. Not just 5 a day, but a rainbow a day . . . your health lies IN that rainbow.

Essentially there are 4 or 5 ingredients in each juice, which tend to be, a mix of fruit and vegetables. Each juice has its own unique use, and its own unique properties. When doing a detox, you will need to follow a plan – a day by day guide that tells you which juices to make and drink each day. These plans are easy to follow, and are devised to ensure that your body receives all of the nutrients it needs, each day, in order to remain healthy. I can recommend the plans of both Jason Vale and Joe Cross, who have both devised the plans with the help of nutritionists.

The "detox" is a great way to kick-start your body into accepting and enjoying healthy food. It is known as a "detox" because you don't put any unhealthy food into your body, so your body eliminates the toxins that are currently residing inside it. At the same time as eliminating those toxins, you are putting nothing but good, healthy foods into your body and therefore replacing bad with good. Your body then becomes used to the good healthy foods and will reject the bad foods.

You hear of celebrities doing a "juice detox" once a month to get rid of the toxins in their body, but life does not work like that. Healthy life is maintained by a complete lifestyle change, not a once a month blast. If you are going to remove toxins from the body, and "kick-start" your body into a healthier way of life, then it has to be a way of life. After your juicing plan, comes healthier eating – 80-90% of your time should be spent eating healthy, and the other 10-20% using freedom mentality for those "special occasions". You will find that after 28 days your body will reject some of the unhealthier foods that you were eating, for instance my body now routinely rejects fatty fried foods, sweets, cakes etc., because I have been fuelling it with the vitamins, minerals and phytonutrients provided by fresh, whole foods. My body has become used to those things and will now accept nothing less.

Some of the side effects of juicing, and especially the healthy eating that follows, include (in my own personal experience): weight loss, the elimination of symptoms of chronic illness (asthma, heart disease, cholesterol etc.), better skin, healthier hair and nails and more – ALL positive! If only the side effects of the drugs we are fed by the medical profession had similar positive side effects, instead of the negative symptom ENHANCING side effects that they do have, in addition to the symptom-INDUCING effects of the processed foods that we eat.

If you wish to try a juicing plan, I would recommend that you begin with 7 or 10 days for optimum effect. If you have a lot of weight to lose, then 28 days is probably a better start point. Will you be hungry? For the first few days, you will – your body will want its usual solid processed foods. It will be getting used to two things: not receiving all of the chemicals and refined foods that it is SO used to getting, and getting used to having food in a different format. After a few days, your body will become used to what you are giving it and as a result will start operating much more efficiently and burning fat.

You will go through periods of withdrawal from the sugars and chemicals that you are used to eating – especially if you drink soda, pop or cordial, lots of coffee, or eat biscuits, cakes, breads etc. During this time, it is very easy to give up and decide that juicing really isn't worth it. You will crave your cola, chocolate, sweets, biscuits, and also foods that you didn't realise contained sugar and the like. You will go through periods of hunger, where you would give anything to eat a huge burger, or a sandwich, or a cooked dinner – do not give up, remember you are doing this for your health, and you will feel better. If you are juicing during winter, then make yourself a warm juice – when we were juicing during January, we made the last juice of the day a homemade soup, delicious warm and filling. If you are looking for something more filling, then the juice plans allow you one "filler" a day – but it has to be healthy. So you can grab a piece of fruit (especially appetite satiaters like papaya, nectarine, apple and banana or some nuts and raisins (non processed) or a whole food bar with nothing but natural chemical free ingredients – check the "free from" or "wholefoods" section of your supermarket or grocery store).

Within 4 or 5 days, your body will get used to it and you will crave processed foods less. Because a lot of the juices have satiaters in them, they are quite filling, once you get used to being filled up by a liquid! I have come to love the colours and the bubbles of oxygen in them. In addition, I love to make up my own juice recipes and experiment with combining different colours and flavours of fruit and vegetables. Also, being a nutritional therapist, I enjoy making up juice recipes geared towards alleviating the symptoms of specific ailments. You will also see that, as a result of all of this change, your body will thank you. Your energy levels will pick up, because your body is not focused on digesting all of the stodge that you are consuming and it does not have to spend time trying to balance the chemicals that you are loading it with. Your mental health will also start to improve and you will feel happier – many of the chemicals in processed foods are addictive and work like other addictive substances, in so far as they make you feel good temporarily and then as their effects wear off your mood drops until you have another "hit". By removing all of this from your body and putting only good in, you will find yourself in a constant plateau of positive mood.

To anyone wanting to try a juice plan, I recommend those in the books by Jason Vale and Joe Cross. You can also get the Jason Vale "SuperJuiceMe" app for your phone or android device, which will guide you through your "kick-starter". Once your plan is over and you wish to continue your juicing, you can download other apps, such as "Juice Pro", which is excellent as it allows you to find a juice by searching ingredient or health condition, and it has lots and lots of juices in there – well over 1000 recipes.

When you get in to juicing, and you have done your "detox", you can devise your own juices, and just drink one or two per day, to keep those essential nutrients going into your body.

Fun In Experimentation

It's great fun to experiment with juices, and why not involve the entire family? The juices that you will have been making and drinking, you will have built up an idea of how they are constructed. They contain a wide variety of ingredients, to ensure that you are getting your RDA of each vitamin and mineral that your body needs to be healthy.

They contain things like carrots, spinach, kale, parsnip, ginger, lemon, lime, orange, berries of all sorts, apples, celery, cucumber, pears, pineapples etc. etc. Jason Vale states that there are two bases for a juice – apple and cucumber and apple and carrot – and if you look at most juices, they will contain an apple and/or a cucumber or carrots. If you use his general rule, then you will never have a bad juice. Start with an apple and two carrots, then add maybe a handful of spinach, a lemon and (what is called a "kicker") a thumb-sized chunk of ginger - this just gives your juice a bit of a kick, and in addition the ginger will help with absorption of the nutrients and helps your digestive system to digest. To an apple and cucumber base, you may want to add a bell pepper, a couple of sticks of celery and some pineapple, with a chilli as a kicker! If you have kids who really aren't sure, then start with what Jason Vale calls "lemonade" – basically an apple or two and a lemon. Then top up with water in order to dilute the strong thick taste of the fresh juice. They will love it. Once they start to ask for it, add a handful of berries, or a carrot and then move on to kale and spinach etc. Use games like "guess the ingredients" or "guess the colour" to make it a bit more fun for them.

Juices are great, because it is an amazing way to get good food into ourselves and our kids, and to be honest, even if you don't like certain fruits and vegetables, when blended together, those you don't like combine with those you do to make new flavours that work for you. I never liked celery, avocado, asparagus, bananas, peppers etc., but I had the juices and didn't even taste them - I now like all of these fruits and vegetables and more that I had never tried, like fennel, chicory, bok choy, persimmon. Juicing has opened up a whole new world for me!

Which Juicer?

Hopefully I have whetted your appetite for juicing, and shown you how it can benefit your health. If you are now planning to do a juice plan, then you will need to purchase a juicer, so here are your options:

Bullet – these are not juicers as such, but more like smoothie makers. You can juice with them, but all of the insoluble fibre remains. It does, however, mash the insoluble fibre, softening it and making it easier to digest. No pulp is produced using this form of juicing. There are studies that show that this is, in fact, the healthiest form of juicing. Contained in the insoluble fibre are certain antioxidants called polyphenols (fibre is known as the polyphenol trafficker), which are required by the gut. When we juice and remove the pulp, we are possibly missing out on these polyphenols or (if they do make it into the juice) they may not make it to the gut and may get absorbed before hand – this is one reason why juicing only (for a longer period than that of a specified plan) is not a great idea – we still need to eat the whole food – fibre and all. . . . juicing is a "kick-starter" for the body.

Price range: £20 - £100

Centrifugal Juicers – These are the most popular form of juicer and most widely available. These juicers produce juice by using a cutting blade to first chop up the produce and then spin the produce at a very high speed. There is a "sieve" beneath that allows the juice to pass through, while keeping the pulp behind. They do produce the juice very quickly and at high speed, but the speed comes from a motor, which can get quite warm and that heat may oxidise and compromise the concentration of nutrients. Centrifugal juicers are also less efficient at extracting juice than single or twin gear juicers, which grind every drop of juice from produce.

Price Range: £50 - £200
Slow Juicers or Masticating Juicers - These juicers have a single gear or an auger instead of blades. The auger basically crunches the fruit or vegetables into pulp,

releasing juice in the process. This crunching process is a highly effective way of breaking down the hard, fibrous cell walls of fresh produce and produces a high juice yield and very dry pulp. Masticating juicers run at a much lower speed but the lower speed produces little heat and therefore minimizes oxidation. That means that most of the vital enzymes and nutrients in your juices are preserved from oxidation since the juicing process doesn't disturb the cellular structure of the produce being juiced. One of the main drawbacks to slow juicing is that, unlike a centrifugal juicer (where you place the whole fruit into the juicer), you have to chop the fruit up into smaller pieces so that they can be put into the machine. Having said that, there are a couple of slow juicers out there – such as the Optimum 600, and Jason Vale's Retro – that will take the whole fruit.

Price Range: £100 - £500

Twin Gear (Triturating Juicers) – these juicers operate like slow juicers, but at a slower speed. They have two augers travelling in opposing directions and the fruit is crushed dry by them, with maximum yield of juice expressed for your benefit. They can juice pretty much every fruit or vegetable you can think of. No heat is produced and therefore the nutrients are safe from any form of oxidisation and are all present for your body to absorb.

Price Range: £750 – a few thousand

Hydraulic Press Juicers – These work in two ways. Firstly the produce is triturated, in terms of being crushed and mashed to a pulp. This pulp is then placed into a muslin bag and the press exerts extreme pressure on the pulp for a full volume juice extraction. These give by far the best quality of juice in terms of nutrient content and yield from the produce used. The pulp is dry and pale, showing not only that all of the juice has been extracted, but also that the nutrients from the produce have also been extracted to their full potential.

Price Range: In the thousands – essential if you want the best quality of juice.

It must be noted here, that items like nuts and seeds, and those fruits and veg low in water content (avocado, banana etc.) should not be juiced, but should be blended into the juice. Ice is also not a substance to put through your juicer.

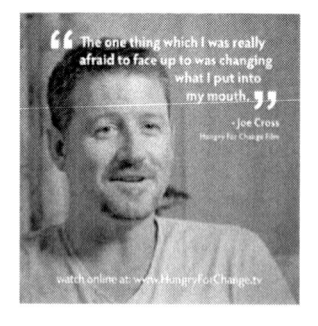

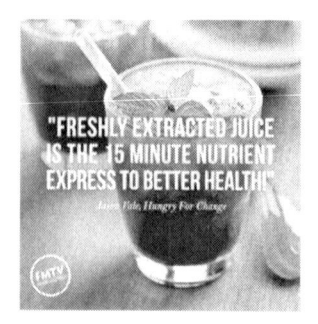

Joe Cross - Watch: Fat Sick & Nearly Dead
Jason Vale - Watch: Super Juice Me

CHAPTER NINE – Time To Be Healthy (or How To Avoid The Doctor!!)

We are now nearing the end of the book, and I have hopefully provided you with many tools in regard to your health and wellbeing – not just for the cells inside your body, but also in terms of physical exercise, mental wellbeing and more. If you have not found anything contained in these pages that you want to implement in your life, or that you have found beneficial in some way, then I hope, at least, that it has provoked thought and discussion within your household or circle of friends.

If the book has excited you and made you spring into action, in order to improve your lifestyle and change your life, then one of the questions that is no doubt on your lips is: What else is there out there that I should not be doing? What other ingredients are contained in things that I should avoid?

In this chapter, I hope to give you a little information that will help you make informed decisions about other non-food related household products. That's right – not only are processed foods unhealthy, but many processed products are. In this chapter we will look at various products that we buy every day, that maybe we should consider replacing with more environmentally friendly, and more importantly, more health friendly products. Those things we use in our daily routines – beauty products, personal hygiene products, cleaning products etc.

With what I have already told you, and your willingness to change these things, and some changes in this area too, you will feel healthier than ever before. By making yourself healthier, and maintaining your new lifestyle (we shall discuss this in the next chapter), you will maintain your health and as time goes on you will become healthier. Your newfound health will also show other benefits too – because you are so healthy, your immune system will be stronger, and you will find that you do not succumb to infections. Great news, huh?

The better news is that this will mean there are no visits to doctors, no unnecessary prescriptions for unnecessary drugs, no unnecessary side effects.
So let's start talking products: (Please bear in mind that all of the following are backed up by scientific academic reports – and that I am in no way trying to scaremonger or stop you from using or buying the products that you use. I am just creating an awareness of the ingredients in those products, the effects that they have on your body and the alternatives that may be available)

*** Personal Hygiene ***

Antiperspirants and Deodorants: These products work to block the sweat ducts or inhibit the growth of bacteria. They routinely contain aluminium compounds in order to do so. Aluminium is known to be toxic to the nervous system and thought to interfere with oestrogen, contributing to the higher incidence of breast cancer. A 2003 study of breast cancer survivors published in the European Journal of Cancer Prevention found that women who began to shave their underarms and use underarm products before the age of 16 had been diagnosed with breast cancer at an earlier age than those who began these habits later. Another ingredient to be wary of is triclosan, which is suspected of disrupting the endocrine system and has been shown to harm the thyroid system.

An alternative to these products is solid crystal deodorant – these can be found in health shops. In addition to the fact that these are 100% natural and just as effective, they have many other benefits – they last for 12 months or more, and they leave no sticky residue meaning you do not get the white tide marks associated with deodorants and antiperspirants. One of the drawbacks to them is that they are more expensive than the everyday products (they cost about 3 to 4 times as much), however when you factor in that you will not need to buy another deodorant stick for 12 months, you are saving around 300% of the money that you would be spending on the products. They are made from a 100% natural crystal called potassium alum, and they work by inhibiting the growth of odour causing bacteria.

Toothpaste – We all use toothpaste, it keeps our teeth clean and means we don't have to have any expensive oral work done. But is your toothpaste good for you? Well, studies show that conventional toothpaste is not really that good for you – it contains a couple of ingredients that have been shown in labs to be carcinogenic. These ingredients are sodium fluoride and sodium laurel fluoride, along with artificial sweeteners. Again, triclosan is likely an ingredient, as it was in antiperspirants, but this time you are ingesting it. Alternatives can be found in your local health food shop – sometimes as organic toothpaste, other times as a tooth powder. We use fennel based toothpaste – when looking for a product like this, it is always wise to check the ingredients list and look for any possible chemicals.

If you want to make your own, that is possible too. You can do something called pulling, where you spend 20 minutes swilling a teaspoon of coconut oil around your teeth, gums and mouth – this is great for overall oral hygiene. In terms of brushing though, as we don't all have 20 minutes a day to spend brushing our teeth – you can use plai n baking soda (or bicarbonate of soda).

You can even brush teeth with plain water, so long as you floss – it's the food that gets stuck in-between your teeth that causes the bad breath, most of the time.

If you want to make toothpaste, try this:
- Half a cup bicarbonate of soda
- 1 teaspoon of fine Himalayan pink salt (NOT table salt – direct application of the minerals in sea salt is good for the teeth – this is an optional ingredient and can be left out if you wish)
- 1 – 2 teaspoons of peppermint extract (or 10 – 15 drops of peppermint essential oil)
- Filtered water – add to desired consistency

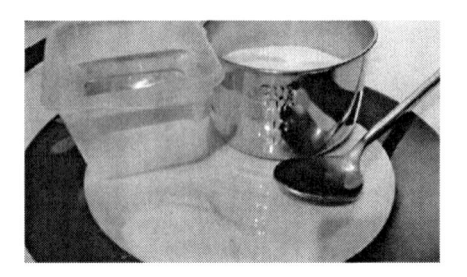

Mix together the first 3 ingredients and then add the water until you reach the desired consistency. Now brush!! Enjoy having clean healthy teeth without using those bad chemicals. If you wish to floss, use unwaxed floss or bee's waxed floss – standard floss is coated with PTFE (used by plumbers on joints to stop leakage and also used in the manufacture of Teflon) which is considered to be carcinogenic.

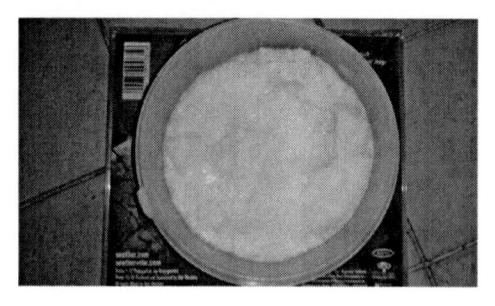

Shower Gels – Shower gels and skin cleansers rely on alcohol and petroleum products to dislodge dirt and clean the skin. These products also, however, remove natural oils and produce skin drying. To counteract this, manufacturers add mineral oils (a petroleum product) to make the skin feel soft. In order to create foam, they will add chemicals such as sodium laurel sulphate, ammonium laurel sulphate, sodium laureth sulphate, ammonium laureth sulphate and myreth sulphate. These chemicals are known skin irritants and may be contaminated with carcinogenic compounds.

Have you ever noticed how certain brands leave your skin itching? That is because the concentration of these chemicals is greater in those products.

Polyethylene glycol (PEG) compounds, such as PEG-7 and PEG-200, are also added to many body washes and cleansers to help them retain water. PEG compounds may be contaminated with ethylene dioxide, a known carcinogen. Common preservatives in cleansers include parabens, which can disrupt the hormone system, and methylisothiazoline and methylchloroisothiazoline, which are immune system toxins. Cleansing creams and body washes may also contain TEA, a skin allergen, potentially toxic FD&C colours, and antibacterials such as triclosan (already discussed). Many also have fragrance, which generally includes phthalates. Phthalates have been linked to reproductive problems.

Although there are many safe and natural alternatives available, always ensure you check the ingredients list first and ensure that there are none of these ingredients in the product you choose. The products available are generally specific to each country, but the best ones are the fully organic unscented variety.

Shampoos & Conditioners – These contain very similar ingredients to shower gels with the same negative effects. Of special concern though are the formaldehyde releasing preservatives such as quaternium-15, DMDM hydantoin, imidiazolidinyl urea and diazolidinyl urea, which are used in many shampoos and conditioners to kill bacteria and reduce the risk of skin infections. Formaldehyde is a known human carcinogen.

There are many commercially available natural and organic shampoos and conditioners, the conditioner using essential oils of various types to condition hair of different manageability.
There are also many natural methods that you can try yourself:

For shampoo, beat 2 large eggs and massage into the scalp, leave on for a few minutes and rinse with warm water. To ensure all egg is out of hair mix 1 cup of warm water with 3 tablespoons of vinegar (dark hair) or lemon juice (light hair), and pour slowly through the hair.

For conditioner, pour 1 cup of warm beer over your hair, and then rinse with warm water. For extra conditioning, a teaspoon of Jojoba oil can be added to the beer.

There are also many other natural recipes for shampoos and conditioners available online, which include the use of banana skins, natural honey and apple cyder vinegar. We are slowly returning back to nature and, when I read some of these recipes, my first instinct is to dismiss them. But then I think about it and realise that thousands of years ago, even hundreds of years ago, our ancestors never had the chemicals that we use today – everything was manufactured from natural ingredients. The fact that we are starting to consider a return to these values is to me an amazing thing and something that I wholeheartedly support.

Cosmetics / Beauty Products

Hair dyes – A study by the Harvard School of Public Health suggested that women who use hair dyes 5 or more times per year are twice as likely to develop ovarian cancer. In 2006 the European Union banned 22

hair dye ingredients, because of their carcinogenic effects. In the USA, these substances are not banned and still used in hair dyes. Other cancers that have been linked to frequent (once every 4 – 6 weeks) use of hair dyes include: bladder cancer, non-Hodgkin's lymphoma, and multiple myeloma. Many hair dyes use coal tar dyes, which are suspected carcinogens. They also contain many ingredients which can cause blindness (in Canada these products have to carry the warning "May Cause Blindness"), skin irritation, endocrine disrupting chemicals and other toxins
The safest alternatives are those which use cassia, henna or indigo and contain non-toxic ingredients. To be totally safe, be happy with who you are and don't dye your hair!! You are awesome, after all!!

Make-up – (Concentrating on make-up that is more frequently used, and applied directly onto the skin or lips, such as eye shadow, lipstick and blusher) The powders used for make-up such as foundations, eye shadows and blushers contain talc, silica or alumina – all three of these are known respiratory irritants when inhaled in powder form. They also contain tar coal dyes for colouring – coal tar dyes are a known carcinogen.

Because these products are worn on the skin for hours at a time, the chemicals that they are made up of are absorbed through the skin and into the blood stream, and can become toxic. The mineral oils used in these products can also clog up the pores and cause acne and black heads. They also contain ingredients which are preservatives and can break down into formaldehyde, another carcinogenic toxin.

The main worry with lipsticks, lip tints and lip glosses is that when tested, 80% were found to contain lead and in other cases other heavy metals like cadmium and arsenic. When you think, an average woman may ingest 4 pounds of lipstick in her lifetime; this is a real concern, as heavy metals are directly linked to cancer. Other ingredients used in lipsticks contain sun screen agents, which when exposed to ultraviolet light break down into free radicals which can affect DNA expression.

Alternatives to lipsticks are those which replace the petroleum wax content with beeswax or olive oils. Again it differs from region to region so keep an eye on those ingredient lists.

Hair Removal Products – Chemical depilatories contain strong chemicals to remove the hair. These chemicals act as skin irritants and because of the strength of the chemicals their effect can be extreme and severe. The high pH chemicals that are used, work by dissolving the hair under the surface of the skin. One of the alternatives used is waxing – these waxes are applied hot, but many manufacturers use petroleum-based compounds in the wax. These compounds contain preservatives which are endocrine disrupting parabens.

There are many alternatives for hair removal, including shaving, but those organic products available will either contain beeswax or no wax at all. Alternatively, you can make your own product: Melt a small amount of beeswax in a small pan, until very warm, but still cool enough to touch. After dusting skin with body powder or corn starch, apply warm wax with a wooden spatula. Allow mixture to cool for a few seconds, and then remove quickly with a light tapping. Soothe skin with aloe vera gel.

Household Cleaning Products

Bleach – Bleach contains sodium hypochlorite as its main ingredient, which is a toxic skin irritant and respiratory irritant. If mixed with vinegar or ammonia (which may be an unlabelled ingredient in some other cleaning products) in turns into chlorine gas which is highly toxic. It may also be a neurotoxin and cause liver disease.

Alternatives include mixing baking soda with tea tree oil and using them as a scrub – tea tree oil is an antibacterial.

Surface Cleaner / Also all-purpose cleaner – Some of these products contain ammonias, which can be strong respiratory irritants, and can also cause kidney and liver damage. They also contain other ingredients, which are neurotoxic, and skin irritants such as butyl cellusolve and ortho phenylphenol.

As an alternative, mix a few teaspoons of tea tree oil with water and use in a non-aerosol spray bottle. Or vinegar cleaner – mix white vinegar 1:1 with water, and use in a non-aerosol spray bottle

Toilet cleaners – These products often contain highly caustic substances, which can cause asthmatic attacks, kidney and liver damage and various carcinogens. These are chemicals like ammonium chloride, dichlorobenzene, hydrochloric acid, and sulphate based ingredients.

As an alternative, use neat white vinegar and scrub to clear lime scale build up, bicarbonate of soda and white vinegar to clear a blockage, or you can pour a can of cola in the toilet! Is this all that it is good for?

Disinfectant – The need for disinfectant is a fallacy, based on a false fear of germs. Normal household cleaning is normally sufficient to eliminate any germs present. The easiest way to remove germs is to use the alternative to bleach as detailed above, plus good old fashioned elbow grease to scrub surfaces clean. Many disinfectants use highly caustic ingredients, such as sodium hydroxide and phosphoric acid, and are a waste of money. Disinfectants should be reserved for hospitals and other places with people with low immune systems.

An alternative to all sorts of household cleaners, is to mix one cup of vinegar to a bucket of water. This can be used for floor cleansing, surface cleansing, glass and mirror cleansing – if you wish to add antibacterial properties then add 15 to 20 drops of tea tree oil to the mixture.

If you stick to using natural products for your health, cleanliness and hygiene, as outlined here, and eating organic natural whole foods, then you should remain in good health and avoid the need to see a doctor. Obviously is you are ill then do not refuse to see a doctor, as there may be something seriously wrong, but you are now more aware of everything that causes the symptoms of illness to appear, and can begin to take steps and precautions to prevent things getting any worse or appearing in the first place. Use your new knowledge to discuss your health with your doctor, and make an informed decision with your doctor's assistance on how to proceed.

"The doctor of the future will give no medicine, but will interest his or her patients in the care of the human frame, in a proper diet and the cause and prevention of disease" - Thomas Edison

CHAPTER 10 – Maintaining The New You

Now that you are (hopefully) on your way to becoming a revolutionised version of your former self – healthy, fit, happy, positive (no matter what) – we need to talk about how you go about maintaining this new you. How do you keep it up? Maintain your willpower? Stay on the wagon? Have you listened to anything I've just said? If you have then you will know. If like some people, you need the odd reminder as to what you are doing and why you are doing it, then I guess this chapter will act as a refresher. If you ever get to the point where you feel like giving up, or you lose your way (as many of us often do) then come back to Chapter 10 and read it, to remind yourself why.

Motivation: You are doing what you are doing, in order to turn your health and your life around, to make a healthier, happier fitter you. In short, you are revolutionising your life!

If you are reading this chapter for the second time, then you are struggling – sit, think and get over it, then continue reading. If you are reading this for the first time, then you are just finishing my book – I hope that you have learnt something that will help you to make your life better; I also hope that you have enjoyed my book, and will read future books; I would like to thank you, sincerely, for purchasing and reading my book and this final chapter should act as a recap of the previous 9.

This book is a lifestyle in 100 or so pages – if you follow the information that I have given in these pages, then your life will change, in ways you never imagined. When a change becomes permanent, a passion develops within the "changee" that keeps the momentum going – sometimes that momentum slows to what seems like a stop and this is when willpower keeps the momentum going.

Remember Will Power is the little fellow sitting on one shoulder, who tells you what's right, and tells the other guy to "get stuffed"!! If you visualise him doing just that, then it will be easy to keep that momentum up, because you will actually become Will, and you will drive yourself to do this right. In order to do it successfully, then you need to be 100% committed to it and believe that this is going to make you healthier, happier, fitter – ***those who believe, achieve!!***

You can use "Freedom Mentality" – do you remember that? But do not ABUSE it – that is, do not use it as an excuse to abuse yourself. If you feel like chocolate or biscuits, a treat, then make sure you do not "feel like" them EVERY day, and that it is a "one off" and a treat. If you remember the 80/20 rule and apply it, then you won't go far wrong. You need to be eating good, fresh, whole foods 80-90% of the time in order to ensure that you are living in a healthy and well body. The rest of the time, it is ok to allow yourself some freedom (this accounts for going out for meals with the family, special occasions like Mother's Day, Birthdays, Christmas etc.), so long as you are straight back onto your healthy foods the next day.

Remember that your lifestyle change will not happen overnight, positive, sustainable changes take time – it can take anywhere from 8 to 18 months in order to attain your goals. In this time though, all of your previous negative habits have turned around to become positive habits, and are now sustainable because your body has become used to your new lifestyle habits. You may get over your addictions to negative lifestyle choices, but every now and then they will creep back to haunt you – after a period of time however, they will no longer bother you.

The choices you make, with regards to your lifestyle, are what make you successful or unsuccessful. Well, if you only make positive choices, then your life can only go one way. All of the advice in this book is given based on my own personal experience, and in order to help you to make the positive choices required to change your life for the better, a few simple rules:

In terms of food, you need to choose fresh whole food over processed or refined foods – for example, if you MUST have sugar go for raw cane sugar over white refined sugar. Go for the food that has minimal human or machine interaction.

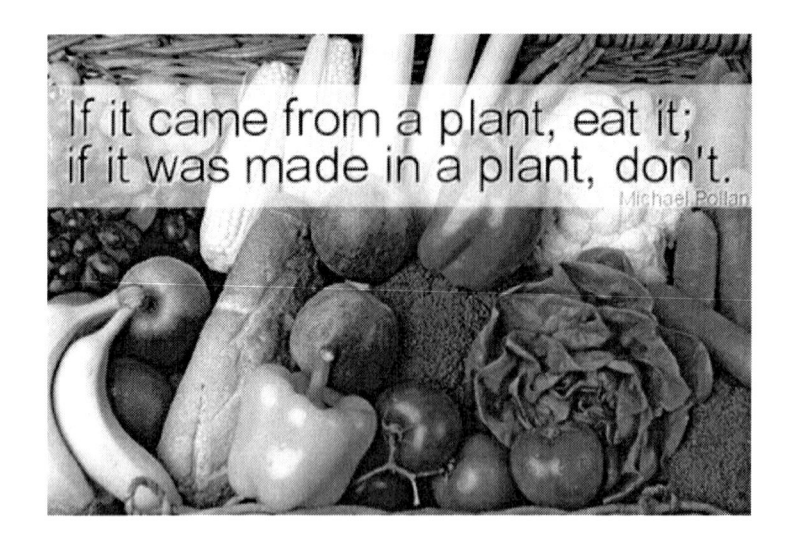

Positive thinking – practice acceptance over resistance – accept that what is meant to be will be, what has passed is past and none of it can be changed. What is to come (the future) can be shaped, but only by what you do today – the NOW. Live in the now, make today affect tomorrow for the better . . . one small change every day is all you need to make in order to move forward and maintain momentum.

Meditate – every day for at least 10 minutes. I have introduced a couple of techniques, and there are many available on YouTube under the search criterion "guided meditation" – listen, learn and practice. Once you have it, you will find that you can do it anywhere (I don't recommend you do it whilst driving though!!) and it helps in all situations – with stress, with focus, with feeling, with meaning. During meditation and at all times, once you get the knack, be mindful of the now.

Try to replace bad foods with good, and set that in your mind as a permanent change. For example - honey in your tea instead of sugar; a bunch of grapes instead of a bag of sweets or a handful of nuts and raisins; or, my own personal favourite, a banana instead of a chocolate bar! If you increase your nutrient intake and decrease your "anti-nutrient" intake (remember C.R.A.P.? Carbonated, Refined, Artificial colourings & flavourings/Alcohol, Processed foods . . . .AVOID AVOID AVOID!!) then you will do just fine, and your palate will adjust, to the point that you will no longer desire those foods that are unhealthy. Healthy foods will become the norm, and you will start to desire them!

Exercise – start with walking, and start small, so a slow walk for 5 minutes each way slowly building up until you are walking quickly, then jogging, then running. With the distance increasing too, from 5 minute to 10, to an hour or longer, before you know it you will be running further and faster than you had ever dreamed – believe me, I know, I've done it. In addition, there are boot camps, exercise classes, gyms, running clubs and more. Exercise is just as important as eating properly – sit still and stagnate, move and metamorphose into a healthy FIT new you. Not only is exercise good for your body, it's also great for the mind – it releases feel good hormone and improves your feelings of wellbeing and makes you feel happy, at peace at the same time as improving your self esteem

Reprogram – this is one of the most important aspects. Things are going to go wrong, and the success of your revolution is dependent upon how you deal with it and your approach to it. If you let it get to you and allow it to bring your mood down, then everything else will fall apart too, *your mind is the concrete holding all of the bricks together.* So when that problem rears its head, remember it's temporary – take a step back, reassess, and reprogram your internal sat nav. All that has happened is that you have taken a wrong turn, hit a dead end or encountered a road blockage of some sort. Reroute around the problem, and continue on your way

to your dream destination – when you reach it, and I promise you will, reprogram for the next dream!!
Every once in a while (I suggest every 4 to 6 weeks) "detox" for 5 days, with liquid nutrients. No freedom mentality, no treats, pure liquid nutrient intake – the original fast food. Get those juicers out and blitz that fruit and veg. You will feel amazing and it will help to reset your new healthy lifestyle, reminding your body and your taste buds (and - from the way it will make you feel – your mind) what healthy eating is all about!
 it's not all about food and drink – remember, the products that you use, not just in terms of beauty products and personal hygiene products but also in terms of household products too, can be just as dangerous (if not more so) as eating those bad foods and drinking those awful drinks

Finally – being healthy is not about being boring. You can still be fun and have fun and be healthy – if people around you can't take the fact that you are being healthy, then change the people or ignore them. People will accuse you of being boring, or not joining in, and try and use peer pressure to get you to eat, drink or do things that you know are going to make you ill, or are unhealthy for you. Don't let it happen – you know the truth – you are the same you, but you are a lot healthier than you were, and you can probably go for longer than your unhealthier friends! Enjoy your new healthy lifestyle – it's awesome, and doing all of this has completely changed me as a person in all ways.

A Story To Finish

Once upon a time, there was a boy, who became a teenager, who became an adult who hated to run. This is the story of a change so substantial that he went from non-runner to running a 10k in just 8 weeks!!! This is the story of one of the greatest achievements of my lifestyle change, and indeed my life.

Every time I am asked to run, or I need to run – well, at least until recently – my reply was from the teenager in me. A loud sigh, a stomp, an exclamation – my boot camp instructor knew that I loathed running. "I don't do running", I would say. This began when I joined boot camp some 7 months prior, when my lifestyle change began.

Then I quit smoking, my alcohol intake reduced, I stopped eating fried, high fat food, I stopped eating and drinking processed high human interaction foods like coffee, refined sugar, sweets, cakes, biscuits etc. and began replacing them with healthy alternatives. Instead of coffee I began drinking warm water with lemon and ginger, and nutritious juices. I started to feel GREAT all of the time every day. My energy levels increased, my positivity increased, my attitude improved – all in all, life improved. I went a step further and removed meat from my diet, becoming a vegetarian – this was also a moralistic lifestyle choice for me too, because of my love for animals.

About 7 months after this all began, I received an email asking if I fancied doing a 10k race in 2 months' time. Having a completely different mind-set and outlook on life, my response was . . . "I can do this" . . . and so I said "YES!!"

I started training immediately, and followed the first step that I stipulated in this book – I found my starting point. After downloading a run tracking app for my phone, I ran 2.5km – a quarter of the distance I was hoping to run. This gave me a time. I then upped the distance to 5km then 7.5km. About half way through my training, on the 4th week, I ran my first 10km and did it in 55 minutes. This was a great time – throughout this time, my self-esteem just kept on snowballing, becoming greater and greater.

My attitude had become – not only can I do this, I can smash my time too!! The biggest motivator was when one of my fellow "boot campers," a guy who had run several 10k races, told me that I would never do it in less than 50 minutes and would be pushed to do it in that – he had never run a 10k faster than 53 minutes he said. So I was determined to beat that – approaching 47 (2 weeks after the race) I wanted to complete the race in a minute for every year, 47 minutes.

I kept pushing myself with every training run, pushing my comfort zone. I was told that the day would bring with it an extra push, in terms of adrenaline. When the day came, I was excited and nervous – I did not want to let myself down, nor disappoint all of those people who had been following my blog for 8 weeks. So the pressure was on.

The race actually was easier than I expected, in the form of adrenaline and an unexpected competitive nature. I wanted to beat all of those around me, who seemed like real "professionals". On the road, each time that I was passed by another runner, I tried to keep up with their faster pace, and once settled into it, I wanted to pass them – and I did on many occasions, they became my pace runners, each time increasing my running pace. My app kept giving me 5 minute updates and my average time got faster and faster, until I ended the race with a nice shiny medal and a time of *46 minutes!!!*

It was such an achievement for me, and I felt so proud of myself!! One of the very best days of my life – I had competed in a 10km race, not only completed it but finished in a competitive time AND in the top 5th of the 1000 entrants. What a day!!

Follow the steps in this book and you too could be achieving things that you always felt were impossible – if you think about it, impossible screams at you *"I'M POSSIBLE"!!* In reality EVERYTHING is possible, if you believe and you have the right focus. Live a life of dreams, revolutionise your life!!

"If you really want to do something, you will find a way. If you don't, you will find an excuse" – Jim Rohn

"In order to succeed, we must first BELIEVE that we can" – Nikos Kazantzakis

"Success is not final; failure is not fatal; it is the courage to continue that counts. Success is a journey, not a destination" – Winston Churchill

CHAPTER 11 – Some Recipes & Tips To Get You Started

Food Recipes

Most of the recipes here are vegan / vegetarian and gluten free – if you wish to make them with meat, then feel free to add some lean organic meat of your choice. Most of the recipes provided courtesy of my lady love.

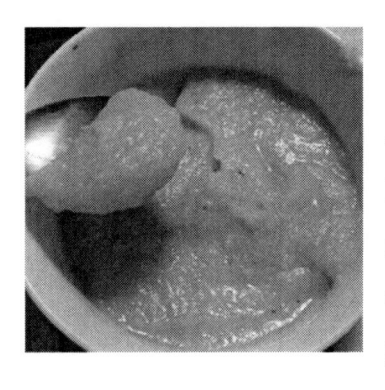

Spiced Parsnip & Apple Soup

Preparation time: 10 minutes

Cook Time: 20 minutes

Serves: 4

Recipe:

- 1 kg parsnips
- 1 Onion
- 1 Medium Bramley Cooking Apple, grated
- 850ml Vegetable stock
- 1 tsp Garam Masala Spice

Method:

1. Peel and chop onion, and fry in a teaspoon of coconut oil
2. Add parsnips, peeled and chopped
3. Add vegetable stock and simmer until parsnips are softened
4. Add grated apple and spice and simmer for a few minutes
5. Blend and serve – season to taste

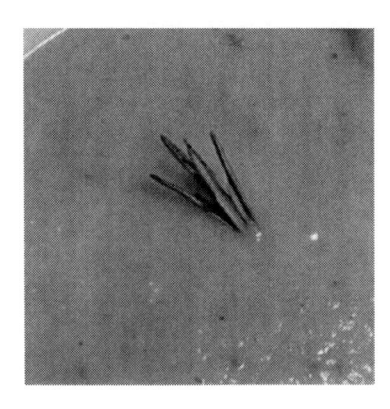

5 Ingredient Cauliflower Soup

Preparation time: 10 minutes

Cook Time: 30 minutes

Serves: 2

Ingredients:

- 1 onion, roughly chopped
- 3 cloves of garlic
- Half a cauliflower, roughly chopped
- 1 tbsp chopped fresh rosemary (or 1 tsp dried rosemary)
- 500 ml vegetable stock

Method:

1. Cook onion and garlic in a tbsp of coconut oil
2. Once onion and garlic are starting to brown, add the cauliflower and rosemary
3. Continue to cook the cauliflower for around 5 minutes, add enough broth to cover the cauliflower, bring to the boil and then turn down the heat and simmer

4. After about 5 minutes, remove the soup from the heat and blend until smooth and creamy
5. Season with Himalayan pink salt and ground black pepper to taste

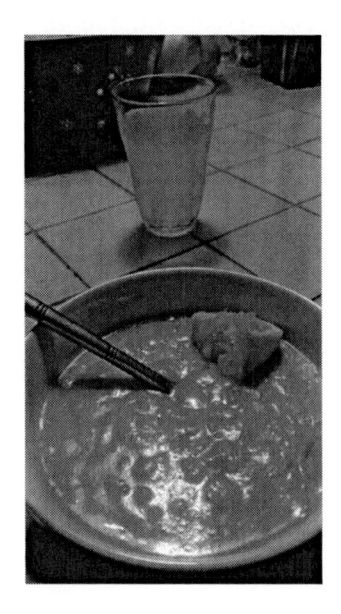

Sweet Coco-Chilli Citrus Soup

Preparation time: 10 minutes

Cook Time: 30 minutes

Serves: 4

Ingredients:

- 2 medium sweet potatoes
- 1 red chilli
- 2 spring onions
- Juice of 1 small lime
- 1 tbsp coconut oil
- 400ml coconut milk

Method:

1. Chop and sauté onions and chilli
2. Peel and chop sweet potatoes into small chunks and add them to the pan, and cook for 5-10 minutes

3. Add remaining ingredients, except lime, and simmer for around 10 minutes
4. Add the juice of a lime, blend with stick blender and serve

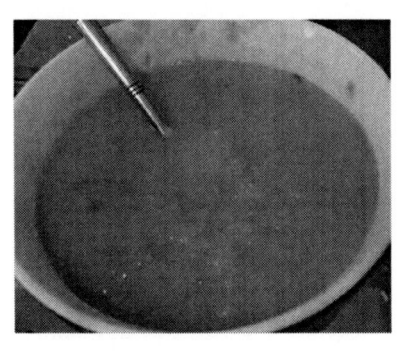

Sweet & Satisfying Soup

Preparation time: 10 minutes

Cook Time: 20 minutes

Serves: 4

Ingredients:

- 750g raw carrots
- 850ml vegetable stock
- Zest of one orange
- 1 orange, peeled & chopped
- 1 sweet onion, peeled & chopped
- 1 stalk of celery
- 2 cloves of garlic
- 3-4 pitted dates (to taste)
- 1 & half inch chunk of ginger root
- 2 tbsp coconut oil
- 1 tsp Himalayan pink salt

Method:

1. Sautee onion, garlic and ginger in coconut oil
2. Add vegetables and stock
3. Simmer for 10 – 15 minutes

4. Whilst simmering zest the orange, then peel and chop. Chop the dates too
5. Add zest, orange and dates and simmer for a further 5 minutes
6. Add Himalayan salt to taste
7. Blend & serve – garnish with pumpkin seeds, hemp seed or fresh coriander

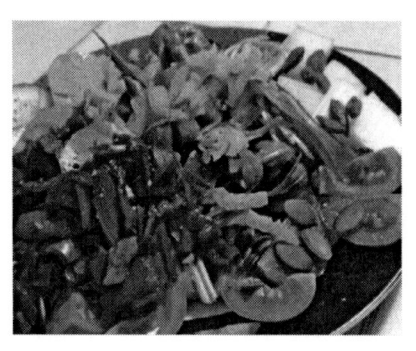

Superfood Salad

Preparation time: 15 minutes

Cook Time: 0 minutes

Serves: As many as you wish

Ingredients:

- Cucumber
- Tomatoes
- Rocket
- Carrot
- Spinach
- Celery
- Goji berries
- Pumpkin seeds
- Red cabbage
- Black pepper (for absorption)
- Baby kale
- Avocado
- Lemon wedge
- Balsamic vinegar

Method:

You can make and eat as much of this as you wish. Shred cabbage and grate carrot. Chop tomatoes, celery and cucumber. Lay all of these on a bed of spinach, rocket and baby kale. Sprinkle with seeds and berries. Season with black pepper and add lemon juice and balsamic vinegar to taste

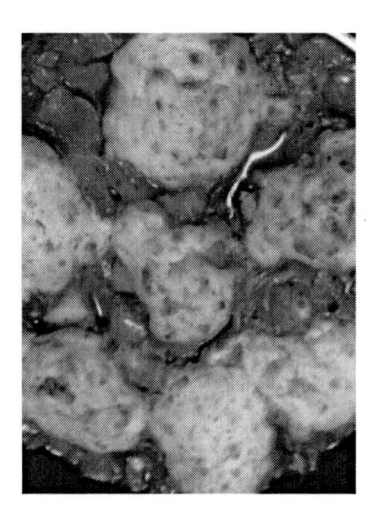

Vegetable Stew & Dumplings

Preparation time: 10 minutes

Cook Time: 50 minutes

Serves: 4

Ingredients: Stew

- 1 tbsp coconut oil
- 1 large red onion
- 1 carrot
- 1 parsnip
- 2 sweet potatoes
- 1 celery stalk
- 1 leek
- ½ swede
- 6 chopped tomatoes
- Fresh parsley chopped
- 1 litre Vegetable stock
- Himalayan salt and black pepper

Method:

1. Heat oil in an ovenproof casserole dish and soften the onion.
2. Add the sliced leek for a couple of minutes and then add the remaining vegetables.
3. Pour on the stock and add fresh herbs and seasoning then cover and simmer for 15 mins

Ingredients: Dumplings

- 200g coconut flour
- 1 tsp baking powder
- 2 tbsp coconut oil, melted
- Dried mixed herbs
- Pinch of Himalayan salt
- 80ml Oat milk

Method:

1. Mix the flour, salt and herbs in a bowl and form a well in the centre.
2. Add the oil and mix and slowly add milk to form a soft dough.
3. If the dough becomes sloppy add more flour.

4. On a floured board split the dough into 8-12 even pieces and roll into balls.
5. Add to the top of the stew and place in the oven without the lid for about 25 mins until golden brown.

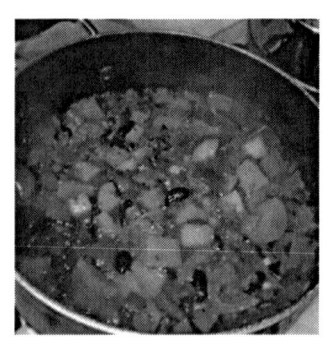

Sweet Potato Chilli

Preparation time: 15 minutes

Cook time: 20 minutes

Serves: 2

Ingredients:

- 2 medium sweet potatoes
- 1 cup of red kidney beans
- 1 courgette / zucchini
- 1 chilli
- 1 red onion
- 1 clove of garlic - crushed
- Zest of orange
- 1 bell pepper
- 2 inch section of turmeric root (or 1 tsp powder)
- 1 tsp oregano
- ½ tsp Himalayan salt
- ½ tsp ground black pepper
- 250 ml vegetable stock

Method:

1. Chop ingredients and add to pan
2. Pour over stock, add kidney beans, orange zest and seasoning
3. Bring to boil
4. Simmer until sweet potatoes are soft
5. Serve

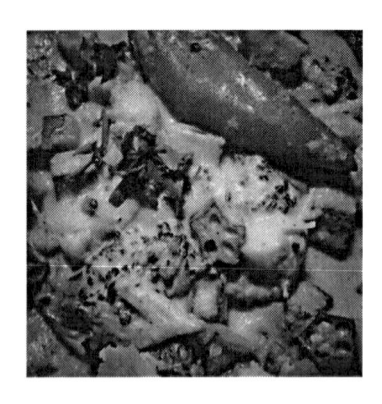

Gumbo Curry

Preparation time: 15 minutes

Cook Time: 40 minutes

Serves: 4

Ingredients:

- 1 tbsp coconut oil
- 1 large onion finely chopped
- 2 garlic cloves, crushed
- 1 tsp turmeric
- 1tbsp ground cumin
- 1 tbsp ground coriander
- 50g cashew nuts, ground
- 400ml coconut milk
- 400ml water
- 175g okra topped and tailed and cut into 1-2 cm chunks
- 250g cauliflower florets
- 250g broccoli florets
- Salt and pepper
- Chopped coriander to garnish

Method:

1. Heat the coconut oil and add the onion, garlic and spices and cook for about 10 minutes.
2. Add the cashews and coconut milk. For a smooth sauce blend at this stage then return to the pan and add the water and simmer for 20mins
3. Steam the vegetables for 5-8 mins, drain and then add to the sauce. Add salt and pepper to taste

Raw Parsnip Rice (served on its own with salad or with your Gumbo Curry)

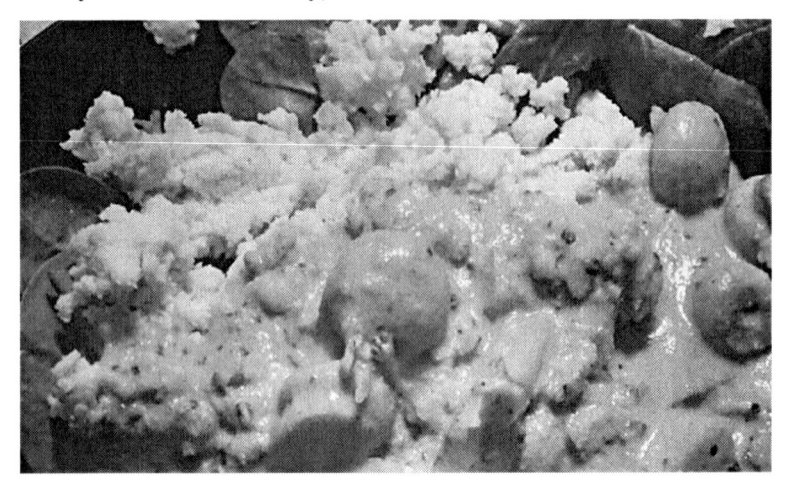

Preparation time: 10 minutes

Cook Time: 0 minutes

Serves: 4

Ingredients:

- 1 parsnip
- ¼ cup ground almonds
- ¼ cup desiccated coconut (soaked in warm water and drained)
- Pinch of Himalayan salt

Pulse in food processor until it looks like rice

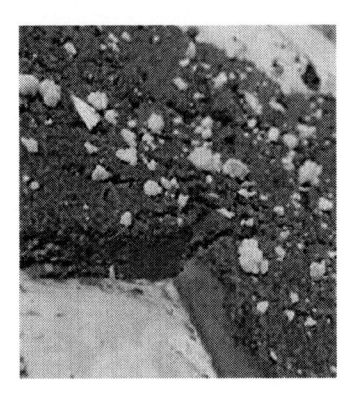

OGP Signature Chocolate Orange Sweet Potato Brownies

Preparation Time: 15-20 minutes

Cooking Time: 25 minutes

Makes: 9-12 depending on how they are cut

Ingredients:

- 2 medium sized sweet potatoes
- Quarter cup raw organic cacao powder
- One & quarter cups of ground almonds
- Quarter cup of raw honey
- Half a cup of pitted dates
- The zest & juice of 1 orange
- Pinch of Himalayan pink salt

Method:

1. Preheat oven to 180 Celsius and line an oven dish with baking parchment
2. Peel, chop and boil sweet potatoes for 5 minutes and then blend until smooth
3. Add all other ingredients and blend

4. Place in oven and bake for 25 minutes or until knife comes out of the finished brownie clean
5. Sprinkle chopped nuts over the brownies before cutting into squares
6. Allow to cool before demolishing!!

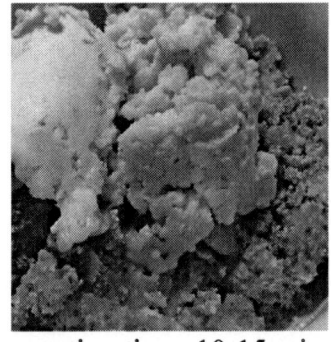

Sweet Potato & Apple Crumble with Homemade Banana Ice Cream

Preparation time: 10-15 minutes

Cooking time: 40 minutes

Serves: 4

Ingredients: Crumble

Filling

- 2 medium sweet potatoes
- 2 large apples
- Juice of orange
- ½ tsp ginger
- ½ tsp cinnamon
- Optional – 1 cup dried fruit

Crumble

- ¾ cup coconut flour
- ½ cup coconut sugar
- ¾ cup oats
- ½ tsp ginger
- ½ tsp cinnamon

- 100 ml hemp oil

Method:

1. Peel and chop potatoes and apples, and put on to boil
2. Whilst they are boiling prepare crumble – combine ingredients in a bowl, and add the oil.
3. Stir to ensure all crumble ingredients are coated in oil and put to one side
4. When apples and potatoes are cooked add spices and orange juice
5. Mash potatoes and apple together and stir in dried fruit
6. Place mixture into an ovenproof dish and cover with crumble
7. Place in oven on 180 C for 20-30 minutes, or until crumble has browned
8. Serve with ….

Banana Ice Cream

Ingredients:

- 3 bananas, sliced

Method:

1. Thinly slice bananas, place on a baking sheet and into the freezer
2. Bananas will freeze quickly (whilst you are eating the main course)
3. Take the frozen banana out of the freezer. Using a food processor or hand blender, blend the frozen banana until it resembles a smooth soft scoop ice cream

Juice Recipes

Remember you can keep a fresh juice refrigerated for up to 24 hours. So if the recipe makes too much for you to drink all in one go, then halve it and put one drink in the fridge for later on or tomorrow. If you freeze it after making it, it will stay good in the freezer for around 3 days.

Allium-Sip - Cold & Flu Remedy

Take at the first sign of cold, then take another 3 days later – symptoms are gone within 24 hours of initial dose, but the second dose makes sure it doesn't come back!!
Ingredients:

- 3 stalks of celery
- 1 red onion
- 1 clove garlic
- 1 spear broccoli
- 1 apple
- 1 inch chunk ginger
- Half a lemon

Process all ingredients in a juicer, stir and drink

Ginger Shot (Energy)

Ingredients:

- 1 apple
- Half inch chunk of ginger

Process in a juicer and drink in one, like a shot – the effects are like those of an espresso coffee!!

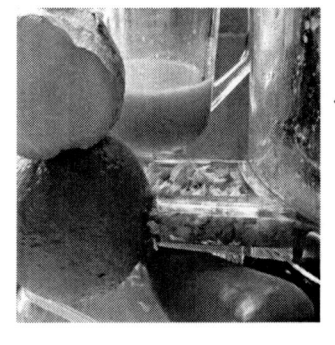

Twisted Firestarter (A shot for the brave)

From Neil Martin – The Natural Juice Junkie www.naturaljuicejunkie.com)

Ingredients:

- 1 small lime
- 1 small chilli
- Half inch chunk of ginger

As with the ginger shot, juice ingredients and drink in one. This one is not for the faint hearted, and on a couple of occasions has initiated the gag reflex. Have a glass of water on hand to take a large gulp from afterwards!!

This one not only has the effect of around THREE espressos, but is also great for the circulation and blood flow and your digestive system, and can also be effective in preventing viruses from entering your body. Good job Neil!!

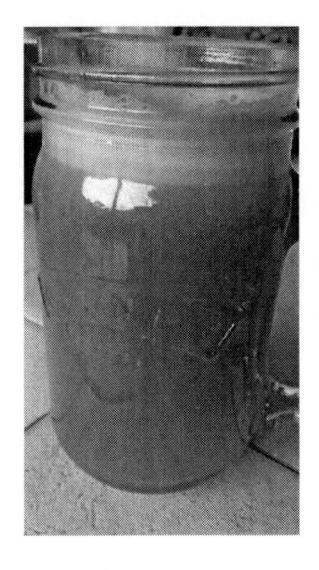

Joe's Mean Green

Joe Cross' Number 1 Juice

(www.rebootwithjoe.com)

Ingredients:

- 1 cucumber
- 4 sticks celery
- 2 apples
- 8 kale leaves (or couple handfuls of shredded kale)
- Half a lemon
- Half inch chunk of ginger

This was the first juice I tried, and it is stunning. Juice the ingredients, and drink. Then feel the goodness start to cleanse your body.

Joe & Neil both have more recipes for you to try on their websites. Once you have a taste for juicing, you will stop at nothing to find new recipes – these websites are jam packed full of them. Once you have the idea, you will be making up your own. As Kat did with the following one!!

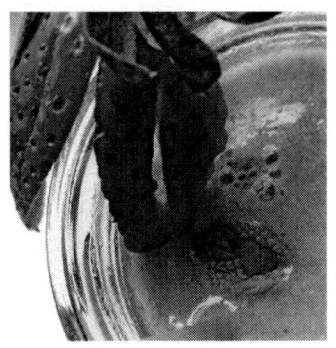

Cupid's Arrow (A Valentine special)
Our cover juice

Ingredients:

- 2 Pomegranate (juice seeds only)
- 2 oranges
- 2 Apples
- 1 lime
- 2 Strawberries & mint leaves to garnish

Juice ingredients, stir, pour, garnish and serve – best to drink with your intended. The thing with our "love juice" is that it is actually good for the heart. Pomegranates are full of antioxidant compounds, but also contain a compound no other fruit contains, called punicalagin. This is shown to benefit the heart and blood vessels. It decreases cholesterol, lowers blood pressure and increases the speed at which heart blockages melt away – so it is great for the blood, circulation and heart.

Other Recipes

Cleaning Fluid – one mug of Apple Cyder Vinegar to 1 gallon of water (to add antibacterial properties to the fluid, add 10-15 drops of tea tree oil) – this is great for cleaning floors, and can be made in smaller quantities to clean surfaces and pet housing too.

Toothpaste –

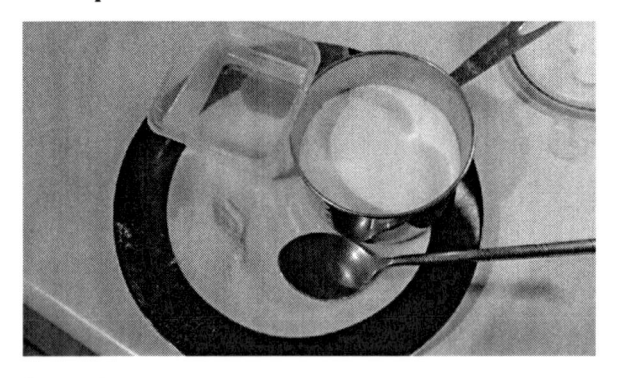

Ingredients:

- Two thirds cup of bicarbonate of soda (baking powder)
- 1 teaspoon of Himalayan pink rock salt
- 1 teaspoon of peppermint oil
- filtered water – to get to required consistency

Method: Mix bicarbonate of soda and rock salt together. Add water until of the desired consistency – a gloopy "paste" that will not run off or through your toothbrush but sit nicely atop it. Finally add the peppermint essential oil, or flavouring of your choice. If you make the mixture too runny, then add some more bicarbonate of soda.

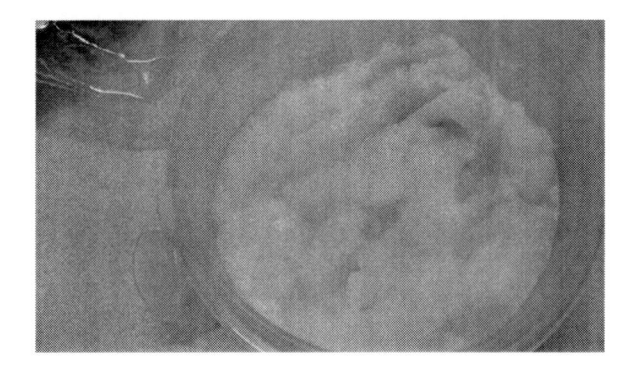

Tips

Sore throats – a mug of warm water, with a slice of lemon, a chunk of ginger and a teaspoon of honey. Drink as often as required throughout the day - much better for you than lozenges or medicines.

Sweet tooth – replace sugar in drinks with honey. Replace sweets with grapes or Inca Berries (Chrysalis).

Quit smoking – celery helps with smoking cessation. Certain chemicals within the celery counteract the craving for nicotine and can help you quit.

Chocolate fiend – When you fancy chocolate, eat a banana, or papaya – these are known satiaters and can satisfy your sweet craving and fill that gap at the same time.

Hayfever – Hayfever is an allergy to pollen. Honey is made from pollen. Local honey is made from pollen in your local area. 1-2 teaspoons of local honey per day can help build immunity to the pollen. Keep it up every day and by next Summer your body should not be affected by the pollen and your hayfever should cease.

Spots – when a spot appears, dab it with organic honey. The honey will work to clear the pore and take away the spot.

Cold sores – take a clove of garlic and cut it in half. Rub the raw garlic onto your cold sore. By the next day it will have gone or be on its way out.

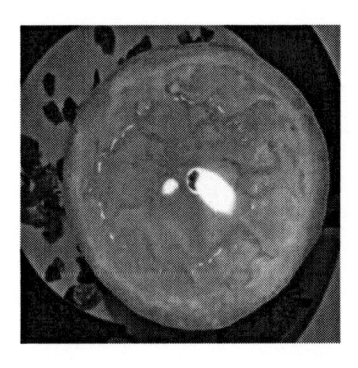

Make your own citrus candle – Score around the centre of an orange or grapefruit. Now score around the pith behind the skin, careful not to go under the central core of pith, gently and gradually peeling the skin away from the meat of the orange. Now twist the skin from left to right, until it dislodges itself. You should end up with half an orange skin, with a central stalk. Half fill the skin with vegetable oil, and light the central stalk – hey presto!! A candle! You will find that it also scents the room.

To see the pictures contained within this book, in their full technicolour glory, and to discover more about me and future publications, please join me on social media:

Facebook: Organic Guinea Pig
Instagram: @organicguinea
Twitter: @OrganicGuinea
@DalePK_Author
Google+: Organic Guinea Pig